Half a Brain is Enough is the moving and extraordinary
little boy who at the age of three was given a right hem
control intractable epilepsy. Antonio Battro, a distinguishe
and educationalist, charts what he calls Nico's 'neuro
humor and compassion in an intriguing book which is p
part meditation on the nature of consciousness and the
manifesto. Throughout the book Battro combines the high
scientific scholarship with a warmth and humanity that
through the intricacies of brain surgery, neuronal archi
application of the latest information technology in educati
is accessible and engaging as well as making a significant
the current scientific literature.

Half a Brain is Enough will be compulsory reading fo
interested in the ways we think and learn.

Born in Argentina, ANTONIO M. BATTRO is a physician and
chologist graduated from the Universities of Buenos Aire
was a fellow of the International Center of Genetic Epist
University of Geneva and an associate director at the Eco
Hautes Etudes in Paris. He received the Guggenheim, Fulb
hower fellowships and was a visiting scholar at the graduat
cation at Harvard University. He has been honored with
National Science award and was an invited lecturer a
Academy of Sciences. He is the author of several book
Piaget: dictionary of terms. He is a member of the Argent
Education.

Cambridge Studies in Cognitive Perceptual Development

Series Editors
George Butterworth (General Editor), University of Sussex, UK
Giyoo Hatano, Keio University, Tokyo, Japan
Kurt W. Fischer, Harvard University, USA

Advisory Board
Patricia M. Greenfield, University of California, Los Angeles, USA
Paul Harris, University of Oxford, UK
Daniel Stern, University of Geneva, Switzerland
Esther Thelen, Indiana University, USA

The aim of this series is to provide a scholarly forum for current theoretical and empirical issues in cognitive and perceptual development. As the twenty-first century begins, the field is no longer dominated by monolithic theories. Contemporary explanations build on the combined influences of biological, cultural, contextual and ecological factors in well-defined research domains. In the field of cognitive development, cultural and situational factors are widely recognised as influencing the emergence and forms of reasoning in children. In perceptual development, the field has moved beyond the opposition of 'innate' and 'acquired' to suggest a continuous role for perception in the acquisition of knowledge. These approaches and issues will all be reflected in the series which will also address such important research themes as the indissociable link between perception and action in the developing motor system, the relationship between perceptual and cognitive development to modern ideas on the development of the brain, the significance of developmental processes themselves, dynamic systems theory and contemporary work in the psychodynamic tradition, especially as it relates to the foundations of self-knowledge.

Published titles include

Jacqueline Nadel and George Butterworth (eds)
Imitation in Infancy

Margaret Harris and Giyoo Hatano (eds)
Learning to Read and Write: a cross-linguistic perspective

Michael Siegal and Candida C. Peterson (eds)
Children's Understanding of Biology and Health

Paul Light and Karen Littleton
Social Processes in Children's Learning

Half a Brain is Enough

The Story of Nico

ANTONIO M. BATTRO

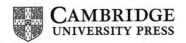

CAMBRIDGE
UNIVERSITY PRESS

PUBLISHED BY THE PRESS SYNDICATE OF THE UNIVERSITY OF CAMBRIDGE
The Pitt Building, Trumpington Street, Cambridge, United Kingdom

CAMBRIDGE UNIVERSITY PRESS
The Edinburgh Building, Cambridge CB2 2RU, UK   www.cup.cam.ac.uk
40 West 20th Street, New York, NY 10011-4211, USA   www.cup.org
10 Stamford Road, Oakleigh, Melbourne 3166, Australia
Ruiz de Alarcón 13, 28014 Madrid, Spain

First published 2000

Printed in the United Kingdom at the University Press, Cambridge

Typeface Monotype Sabon 10.5/14.5pt.   *System* QuarkXPress™   [SE]

A catalogue record for this book is available from the British Library

ISBN 0 521 78307 0 hardback

For Ellen Winner and Howard Gardner

Contents

Preface

This is a short book about a long personal story about the brain, the mind, and education. It began some forty years ago when I received my degree as a physician from the University of Buenos Aires. After training in electroencephalography and neuroanatomy I won a scholarship from the University of Paris to do experimental research in perception with Paul Fraisse. After my doctorate in psychology, while I was taking courses in mathematical logic and philosophy at the University of Fribourg, Jean Piaget invited me to Geneva. I spent two years with Piaget as a fellow of the International Center for Genetic Epistemology. At that time I met Seymour Papert who was doing research on artificial intelligence with Marvin Minsky. Twenty years later at MIT he started a revolution in education with the computer language called Logo. I was then rapidly introduced to the humanitarian use of computers with handicapped children and returned to work in Buenos Aires with the deaf. With my student, and now my partner, Percival J. Denham, we began to extend new information and communications technology to a wider population of physically and mentally disabled children. In a few years of intensive work and travel we shared our expertise in many South American countries, particularly in Argentina and Brazil, where we gradually established the practice not only of clinical computing for disabled persons, but of a more inclusive digital education for all.

Then one day a five-year-old boy came to our laboratory to be introduced to the new digital environment of computers and networks. This book is about Nico, an exceptional child who, two years prior to our meeting, had undergone a right hemispherectomy because of severe and intractable epilepsy. There are about one hundred people in the world with this condition, but each one is unique. This particular boy became my friend and my pupil, started school successfully and is now enjoying the fast-growing new world of knowledge. I am privileged to work with him. He has changed my views on the brain, education, and mental development. I thank him daily for the unique opportunity he has given us to learn more about ourselves, most especially that there is no such thing as half reasoning with half a brain.

Finally, I must heartily thank Harvard University for inviting me to be a visiting scholar at the Graduate School of Education and my friend Howard Gardner who encouraged me to write this book. His comments and critiques and those of my friends and colleagues: Fernando Vidal, Kurt Fischer, Thierry Deonna, Marvin Minsky, Balázs Gulyás, Jacques Vonèche, and Ralf Kockro, have helped me to follow the two interwoven threads of the book: the case history of a hemispherectomized child and the neurocognitive roots of education. I also thank Patrick Temple for his assistance with the English version of this text. My thanks also to Sarah Caro, my editor at Cambridge University Press, and to Steve Caro, the most able corrector.

For reasons of privacy I cannot mention the names of the family, teachers' and friends who are involved in making Nico's life worth living, but the reader can imagine my enormous debt to them all. They have kindly supported my passionate research into the best possible education for a bright mind with half a brain.

Glossary

Agents   Elementary mind processes which perform simple actions and can interact in complex patterns. Agents are easy to understand while their interaction could be more difficult to explain (Minsky, 1986).

Brain images   Slices of the brain by X-ray computer tomography (CT), positron emission tomography (PET), magnetic resonance imaging (MRI) and functional magnetic resonance imaging (fMRI). Brain images with better temporal precision require event related potentials (ERP), electrocorticography (ECo), electroencephalography (EEG), and magnetoencephalography (MEG).

Catastrophe theory   Mathematical theory that models some unstable dynamic system where a small local perturbation can produce large global changes. It has been used in biology and psychology to describe and predict sudden and qualitative changes in form and behavior (Thom, 1972).

Cognitive illusion   A bias of some intuitive judgments that are unreasonable but compelling (Tversy & Kahneman, 1982).

Compensatory analysis   The study of the brain processes supporting a specific reorganization of behaviour.

Connection prism   Elementary set of nodes and links that relate persons, machines (computers) and environments. The *World Wide Web* is a very large collection of connection prisms.

Cortical shift   The substitution of one area of the cortex by another during action or thinking. This happens, for instance, when the computer is operated with vocal commands instead of the hands in order to make a drawing. A cortical shift from the hand to the language area induces a new skill in the latter.

Cyclopean vision   A central visual process that extracts information which is hidden when the visual stimuli are viewed monocularly. For instance a pattern of random dots may convey no significant information to the retinas but it can be fused at a higher cortical level and show a figure against the random background (Julesz, 1971).

Digital shift   The change from the analog to the digital, from the continuous to the discrete. It happens, for instance when we make a click with the mouse.

Fractals   Fragmented and irregular objects implying *scaling*, i.e. their degree of irregularity and/or fragmentation is identical at all scales (Mandelbrot, 1982).

Epigenesis   In biology the term is related to the development of the embryo in a sequence of gradual diversification and differentiation of tissues from the initially undifferentiated zygote; in developmental psychology it suggests a qualitative transformation in the organization of our actions and thoughts during growth and implies novelty and creativity.

EQ, encephalisation quotient   The ratio between the actual brain size and the size expected for an animal of equivalent body size (Jerison, 1979).

Genetic epistemology   The study of the formation of knowledge and of the cognitive relations between the subject and the objects. It is not to be confused with genetic psychology which seeks within the study of the child the solution of general problems (intelligence, perception, etc.) and is not identical with child psychology, which is the study of the child himself (Piaget, 1949, Battro, 1973).

Hemianopia   A partial loss in the visual field. In the intact brain the visual information from the right retinas (left visual field) of both eyes travel through the optic nerve, optic tract and optic radiations to the primary visual cortex in the right hemisphere, and signals from the left retinas (right visual field) go to the left hemisphere. In the case of a right hemispherectomy there is a loss of the left visual field: a left (homonymous) hemianopia.

Hemiplegia   Paralysis of one half of the body following an injury of the motor areas and pathways in the brain.

Hemispherectomy   A surgical intervention that removes the cortex of one hemisphere of the brain. In the case of a functional hemispherectomy some of the nervous tissue remains in situ but is entirely disconnected from the rest of the brain.

IQ, intellectual quotient   The ratio between the mental age, measured by psychometric tests, and the chronological age (multiplied by 100). The Wechsler Intelligence Scale for Children, or Wisc measures a verbal IQ and a performance IQ.

Intellectual prosthesis   Computer devices and software that provide assistance to some impaired cognitive processes in speaking, drawing, writing, learning, and perceiving.

Intrinsic geometry   An example is the "turtle geometry" of the computer language Logo where complex geometric objects can be produced using few and simple local commands like Forward, Back, Right, Left, Pitch, Roll and Veer without the need of external coordinates (Papert, 1980, Reggini, 1985).

Lesion analysis   A methodology that correlates a specific region of a damaged brain with changes in a particular behavior (Damasio & Damasio, 1989).

Multiple intelligence theory, MI   The human mind shows at least eight separate modules or faculties called intelligences: spatial, logical-mathematical, linguistic, naturalist, musical, bodily-kinesthetic, interpersonal, and intrapersonal (Gardner, 1983, 1999).

Mental organ   Equivalent of a physical organ in the mental realm. For Noam Chomsky the mental organs are genetically determined, as is the case of language. His view is opposed to the constructivist theory of Jean Piaget concerning knowledge and language (Piatelli-Palmarini, 1994).

Neuroeducation   The theory and practice of the neurocognitive sciences in the field of education.

Neurophilosophy   A theory that views philosophical problems in the light of the new facts and models proposed by the neurocognitive sciences, in particular that the mental processes are brain processes (Churchland, 1989).

Preformation All the parts of an adult organism are contained in miniature in the germ cell. It is the opposite view of epigenesis and excludes innovation, also in the psychological sense.

Split brain The result of a section (or absence) of the fibers connecting one hemisphere to the other (corpus callosum and other commissures). In the split brain condition the individual may show a disconnection between the cognitive activities of the two hemispheres (Gazzaniga, 1970).

Skill A capacity to act in an organized way in a specific context (Fischer and Bidell, 1998).

Stage A state of stable equilibrium during mental development. The stages are necessary steps during the child's growth process and were described by Jean Piaget in four periods: sensory-motor, pre-operational (symbolic, representational), concrete operational and formal operational (Piaget & Inhelder, 1963).

Termites A name given to the gifted and talented subjects studied by Lewis M. Terman (1925–59).

Virtual reality A digital three-dimensional dynamic representation of any environment or object that allows exploration, interaction, and search.

Virtual brain A digital three-dimensional representation of a real brain, useful to study and simulate brain surgery on the computer.

The heart is in the brain

ubi enim est thesaurus tuus ibi est et cor tuum

For where your treasure is, there will your heart be also

MATTHEW, 6:21

This is a book about education and human nature. I would like to share a personal experience about our brains, mine and yours, so as to open up a debate about the brain, education and human development from a new perspective: that of brainpower and brain efficiency. In a sense, this book is an attempt to become aware of the treasure we have inside our skull, "for where your treasure is, there will your heart be also." And the heart is in the brain.

The expression "the heart is in the brain" is not simply a metaphor, it can be interpreted literally from the point of view of modern neurology, as described by Antonio R. Damasio (1994):

> there is a region of the human brain, the ventromedial prefrontal cortices, whose damage consistently compromises, in as pure a fashion as one is likely to find, both reasoning/decision making, and emotion/feeling, especially in the personal and social domain. One might say, metaphorically, that reason and emotion "intersect" in the ventromedial prefrontal cortices, and they also intersect in the amygdala.

And the author continues,

> there is a region of the human brain, the complex of somatosensory cortices in the right hemisphere, whose damage also compromises

reasoning/decision making and emotion/feeling, and in addition, disrupts the process of basic body signaling. (p.70)

But we shall see that when the right hemisphere is anatomically or functionally removed, as in the case we are going to discuss, the remaining hemisphere compensates actively for the loss and no major problems in cognition, sociability, and emotion appear.

New clues have emerged from this study of a child with congenital hemiplegia who was subjected to a right functional hemispherectomy because of intractable epilepsy at the age of three years and seven months. This child, Nico, has lost the use of an entire hemisphere but goes to school, where he has been closely studied from kindergarten to third grade. These three years in particular (five to eight), though only a short span of time, are so very important in a child's life. Moreover, I consider this research to be the start of a longitudinal study which should be continued until early adulthood. It will hopefully give me the opportunity to work on the foundations of a new field, to which I propose to give the name "neuroeducation," with the purpose of bridging the gap between the science of education and the neurosciences.[1] I shall also try to show how to empower the brain (or half of it) with the "prosthetic" use of computers and how this might relate to the global distribution of knowledge in the new digital society. It is an ambitious program but I am certainly not alone in this voyage of discovery.

This book might also be used as a tentative guide to the education of a half-brained child. It would give me great satisfaction if it could help those families in which someone has undergone the ordeal of radical surgery, such as a hemispherectomy. But I must stress the fundamental point that Nico's remarkable rehabilitation is partly due to the fact that the hemispherectomy was performed on his minor right side at an early age. If the same operation were to be performed on the dominant left hemisphere at a later age, the overall result might be different, and certainly not always as satisfactory as in the case we shall discuss here at length. This book is therefore based on the fortunate case of a left half-brained child and should not be extrapolated to other cases without due distinction.

I shall try to show how the scientific study and tender care of a single half-brained child might shed new light on the understanding of the universals of human nature. The opportunity to work with Nico has changed my intellectual life, and has certainly enriched my affective experience. This remarkable, intelligent, and affectionate boy has challenged most of my ideas concerning the brain, the mind and the computer, and may possibly also shake up some of yours. I can better understand now the profound impact that some pupils can make upon their teachers or some patients upon their doctors. Such unique cases produce a change in our views about man. Nico is certainly one of these privileged persons and I am deeply indebted to him.

Medicine is rich in studies of extraordinary neurological cases. The one-case style became popular in our time thanks to the writing talent of distinguished physicians such as Alexander R. Luria (1972, 1986, 1988), Oliver Sacks (1987, 1995, 1997), Norman Geschwind (1987), and Antonio R. Damasio (1994). Some patients have been monitored for decades, like "the man with a shattered world" reported by Luria after thirty years of observation. Psychology too has a long history of one-case reports. Jean Piaget was certainly a master of the detailed developmental analysis of individual children. He published his celebrated research on his children, Laurent, Jacqueline and Lucienne, in three complementary books: *La naissance de l'intelligence chez l'enfant*, Piaget (1936); *La construction du réel chez l'enfant*, Piaget (1937) and *La formation du symbole chez l'enfant*, Piaget (1945). I have a nice story to tell. The first time I had the pleasure of lunching with my "patron" at his house in Pinchat, near Geneva, Madame Piaget, née Valentine Chatenay, a psychologist by training, told me that she always wore a tiny notebook attached to her necklace so that she could record her observations of their children. These careful reports contributed substantially to her husband's research. To this maternal and paternal dedication I would add Luria's (1986, p. 147) comments: "romantics in science want neither to split living reality into its elementary components nor to represent the wealth of life's concrete events in abstract models that lose the properties of the phenomena themselves. It is of the utmost importance to romantics to preserve the wealth of living reality, and they aspire to a science that retains this richness."

A permanent record of our beloved Nico's works and deeds at school is also kept by his teachers. I do not keep an equivalent register at home, but his parents regularly share the most significant developments with me. What I appreciate most is the loving care and commitment which support a long-term observation, an attitude that has more in common with "romantic" science than "classic" science, to use Luria's terms. In sympathy with the values of romantic science my friend Thierry Deonna, an expert child neurologist, wrote to me, "an accurate neurological, scientific description of deficits, compensatory strategies, etc. is perfectly compatible with a description of the 'roman de vie' in which such a unique experience unfolds and which gives it its proper existential dimension."[2]

As for the medical aspects of the surgery known as functional hemispherectomy, (I use the term hemispherectomy as a synonym for hemidecorticectomy or hemidecortication), this clever technique was conceived and executed by the neurosurgeon Jean-Guy Villemure and his team at McGill University to solve the problem of intractable epilepsy. The essential details on functional hemispherectomy are given in Tinuper *et al.* (1988), Smith *et al.* (1991), Villemure and Rasmussen (1993), Villemure and Mascott (1995). They have devised a new way of removing the damaged brain hemisphere without risk of a neurological catastrophe. Instead of producing a whole and complete anatomical recession of the hemisphere, which might have devastating effects, they successfully tried a more physiological intervention. This functional surgery increases the chances of a successful rehabilitation following the removal of a significant part of the brain. In particular, it inhibits hemosiderosis (iron deposit in cells) and hydrocephalus, the most serious problems in anatomical hemispherectomies. Recent statistics show that most patients react very positively to this intervention, the seizures disappear and cognitive functions can even be enhanced.

Nico suffered a congenital left hemiplegia, but managed to walk before he was one year and seven months old and started to speak in sentences shortly before his second birthday. The first two epileptic seizures happened when he was a twenty-two months old, but they then completely disappeared during the following eight months, at which point they recommenced, with repeated convulsions and loss of consciousness. Medication proved useless and a dramatic increase in epileptogenecity was observed. An EEG confirmed an extended epileptic focus in his right cortex involving the right temporal, frontal and parietal area. Finally, when Nico was three-years-and-seven-months old the family decided to try a neurosurgical treatment. The operation was originally to be restricted to a limited resection of the right temporal lobe and a disconnection of the right frontal lobe under corticographic control. However, after the first ablation and disconnection had been performed the corticography continued to show multiple spikes and discharges in the remaining right areas. The physicians discussed the options with Nico's parents and they agreed to a functional hemispherectomy being completed. The technique applied in this case consisted of the removal of the central cortical region, the parasagittal cortex and cingulate gyrus, plus a complete temporal lobectomy, including amygdala and hipoccampus. The remaining portions of the frontal lobe and parieto-occipital lobes were also disconnected from the brain stem and the opposite hemisphere. The pathology found was polymicrogiria of the right temporal and parietal lobes with mild chronic meningitis. Nico made a remarkable recovery. The seizures disappeared, he never lost his speech and in a few days he started to walk. He is now a healthy boy and a good pupil at school. The amazing fact is that nobody would imagine this impressive neuronal loss from his overt behavior. Indeed without seeing his brain images it is impossible to believe that Nico has only half a brain left! Figure 1.1 shows a dramatic view of this functional right hemispherectomy.

In order to take a further step inside Nico's remarkable left brain we could use other kinds of imaging technologies, such as functional magnetic resonance images (fMRI). But I still consider that some experimental research with non-invasive brain technologies is simply not justified, even with volunteers. I believe in the classic dictum: primum non nocere, even if the fMRI does not hurt. I am sure that these technologies will improve significantly in the near future, not only in image resolution but in friendliness, and the time will come to proceed further in our description of the function of this particular half-brain. To sum up, it is difficult to correlate the "catastrophic" reduction of his gray matter with Nico's normal cognitive, social and affective development. His only apparent problem is that he limps and cannot easily move his left arm. He also has a left hemianopia and has difficulty focusing on a visual target, for instance when reading, but in some tasks, such as spoken and written language, he is at the top of his class. How is this possible? How can half a brain sustain a full mind?

(a)   (b)

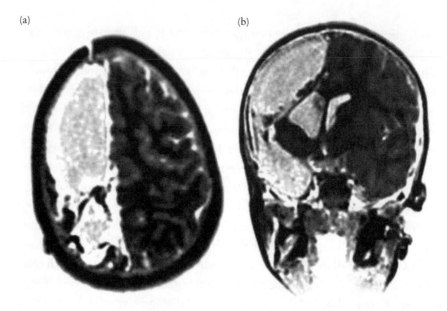

Figure 1.1   Two images of the functional right hemispherectomy. (Nico: three-
years-and-seven-months): (a) horizontal (axial) view, (b) frontal
(coronal) view. Only the left hemisphere is seen, most of the right hemisphere has been removed.

In order to answer this question it is important to take a general view of the
problem. Hemispherectomy or hemidecortication are extreme surgical inter-
ventions in medical practice, and most of the publications on the subject are
clinical reports, follow-ups and statistics from neurosurgeons or neurologists. I shall not deal here with the medical aspects because there are several
good reviews which may be consulted.[3]

It is, however, interesting to note that hemispherectomy has not stimulated
as much fundamental neuropsychological research as split brain surgery has.
While the psychological literature on brain bisection is still growing, the
study of the cognitive, affective and social consequences of the excision of a
brain hemisphere is insufficient. This book is, in a sense, a modest attempt to
enrich our psychological and educational knowledge of the consequences of
hemispherectomy, but certainly much more should be done. In fact, neuropsychologists are somehow late-arrivals in the field. Previously the central
question concerned brain laterality and dominance. Now, and I think this is

progress, the problem is shifting to compensatory neural strategies and to the related questions of brain efficiency and capacity.

We can start with a landmark in the new philosophy of the brain. The philosopher Karl R. Popper and the neuroscientist John C. Eccles, in their classic book *The Self and Its Brain* (1977) have analyzed the left and right excision of the hemispheres. They reported that while the complete removal of the dominant (left) hemisphere gives somewhat enigmatic results, "the excision of the minor [right] hemisphere under local anesthesia gives rise to no loss of the patient's consciousness or self-awareness." And from that crude observation the authors reached the bold conclusion that a "minor hemispherectomy gives a result in complete agreement with the postulate that self-consciousness is derived only from neural activities in the dominant [left] hemisphere" (pp. 330–2). They concluded that the right hemisphere was a "minor brain." The clinical observations of Obrador (1964) and Austin, Hayward and Rouhe (1972) had already articulated this idea. Some years later, Michael C. Corballis (1983) analyzed the cognitive consequences of early and late surgical removal of the left or right hemispheres, the so-called Margaret Kennard doctrine: "the earlier the brain damage occurs the less the behavioral loss." The time at which a brain injury occurs is essential to the making of predictions and taking medical decisions. A detailed overview of the onset of the brain lesion and its impact on mental development can be found in Elizabeth Bates (*et al.* 1992). The issue being examined was the extent of brain plasticity in children and adults, in particular the recovery of linguistic skills in the absence of the dominant hemisphere. At that time the mortality rate was very high in this kind of neurosurgery, especially in adults, and it was difficult to make sound comparisons between left and right excisions. But, nevertheless, neurologists reported an amazing capacity for recovery of language after the removal of the left cortex. Thus the study of hemispherectomized subjects became an important issue in the debate on hemispheric equipotentiality and language acquisition.

The concept of "hemidecorticate syntax" was introduced. In a study of ten children subjected to left or right hemispherectomy because of infantile hemiplegia, Maureen Dennis (1980) discovered that left and right hemispheres "perform different encoding and decoding operations on a syntactically complex sentence in order to identify its meaning". In particular, left hemispherectomized children were inferior to their right counterparts in both "ease and speed of syntactic discrimination, despite their similar verbal and non verbal intelligence." The results of Dennis and Kohn (1975) on nine cases of infantile hemiplegia who underwent left or right hemidecortication show that some syntactic skills, such as the comprehension of passive negative sentences of the kind "the truck was not hit by the car," were inferior in the left hemidercorticates compared to the right hemidecorticates. For example, Dennis and Whitaker (1976) have shown that one left hemidecorticated and two right children who underwent surgery prior to the age of five months, confirmed this linguistic asymmetry as "an organizational, analytical, syntactic problem, rather than a difficulty with the conceptual or semantic aspects of language." In research on written language acquisition after hemispherectomy Dennis (1981) has analyzed how the isolated hemisphere learns to read, write and spell in different ways. We shall discuss this most important topic later and also some new opportunities for using computers to enhance writing skills in the "atypical" brain – as Dennis called it – of a right hemispherectomized child. There were scarcely any computers at school twenty years ago and at that time the radical change which can be affected at the cortical level by computer word processing was unimaginable!

Research on speech and language in hemispherectomized children and young adults still continues to dominate the interest of neuroscientists. The work of R. E. Stark and associates (1995, 1997) provides a good example of the "left to right" transfer of language processes in left hemispherectomized subjects, but there are few studies about the inverse transfer of cognitive processes from the right to the left hemisphere. Perhaps the best analysis of the cognitive consequences of hemispherectomy is to be found in the review by Faraneh Vargha-Khadem and Charles E. Polkey (1992). The authors are aware of the lack of cross control of several variables in most studies (and they analyze fifty-one recent papers), such as age of initial disorder, age of hemidecortication, time elapsed since surgery, and psychological testing, left- or right-handedness before surgery, etc. They conclude that for those subjects with a left hemispherectomy

> a) the isolated right hemisphere has a basic visual and auditory lexicon consisting of concrete and high-frequency words; b) the isolated right hemisphere can recognize, comprehend, and produce words from this

lexicon through both speech and writing; c) in contrast with these domains of ability, the isolated right hemisphere has difficulty comprehending abstract, low-frequency and low-imagery words, manipulating subtleties of grammatical structure, and analyzing words according to their phonetic features. (p. 144)

Nothing particularly relevant is said of the right hemispherectomized subjects except that, "contrary to expectations, no gross deficits on many visual tasks sensitive to right hemisphere function, such as spatial orientation, visuospatial construction and face perception" were found (p. 146). Only one case of prosopagnosia – a cognitive deficit in human face recognition – was reported by Sergent and Villemure (1989) in a thirty-three-year-old patient who had undergone a right hemispherectomy at the age of thirteen following seizure onset at the age of five.

It is interesting to note that there are no reports of serious language impairment in right half-brained children or adults. This makes sense if we accept that language has a left brain location in most right-handers but we also know that there is a significant percentage (70 per cent) of the population of left-handers that may have a bilateral cortical representation of language as reported by Satz (1979). Unfortunately, we lack statistics on the number of left-handers among the right hemispherectomized population to make a comparison. The question of the different cognitive outcomes of right and left hemispherectomy is still a matter of discussion. Our study is about a right-handed boy with a high linguistic performance, but in scientific literature the focus continues to be the loss of the left brain, not of the right one, as in our case study.

The core of the debate was again correctly identified by Corballis (1983):

> at one extreme we have the notion of two hemispheres as fundamentally the same and as interchangeable, but each programmed differentially by different rates of growth on the two sides. At the other extreme, we have the idea of the hemispheres as fundamentally different, each predestined to develop its own specialized functions. The one extreme emphasizes symmetry, continuity between humans and other species, and plasticity of function; the other stresses asymmetry, discontinuity, and rigid predetermination. Perhaps by keeping these extremes in mind, we shall be able in the future to arrive at a correct compromise. (p. 110)

I think we are closer now to reaching a new synthesis. The decisive factor might be the introduction of non-invasive dynamic brain image technologies, such as positron emission tomography (PET) and functional nuclear magnetic resonance images (fMRI). The impact of the new imaging techniques as a research and clinical tool is enormous. A good introduction to the non-invasive technologies is the splendid book *Images of Mind* by Michael I. Posner and Marchus E. Raichle (1994) and publications by Bigler (1996), Damasio (1995), and Salamon (*et al.*, 1990). It is important to note that the first dynamic brain images performed by Pawlick (*et al.*, 1990) on patients who had undergone hemispherectomies because of uncontrollable epilepsy show a remarkable involvement of association areas in both motor and speech activation. This new frontier of knowledge should be explored, but before proceeding any further, a careful and explicitly ethical approach is needed in case a conflict occurs between the interests of the patient and the advancement of science. The beginning of a promising new field of research often implies new moral dilemmas.

We may now return to our main question. How can half a brain sustain a full mind? And this in turn leads us to the brain/mind controversy – a very difficult epistemological problem that should be solved some day. New laboratories and research departments are being dedicated to the neurocognitive sciences and in several countries new journals contribute to the advancement of the field. We will rapidly globalize the findings through the Internet, where some leading scientists are now sharing interactive brain models on the Web. The number of scientists, publications, meetings, and grants in the neurocognitive sciences is rapidly increasing and I am convinced that only collaborative work on an international scale will succeed.[4]

Let us start with the most basic knowledge about the evolution of the nervous system. Evolutionary theories tell us that the mind and the brain evolve together, and as Harry Jerison (1979) affirms, "the size of the brain, its weight or volume is an extraordinarily useful measure in neurobiology." But the problem is that nobody can explain why *Homo sapiens sapiens* have such a huge brain if it can be shown that, following surgery, half of this brain suffices! The once famous, encephalization quotient (EQ), and the ubiquitous intellectual quotient (IQ) are, in my opinion, two mismeasures of the mental capabilities of man, in particular in the case of hemispherectomized individuals.

For a very well founded critique on the IQ, where intelligence quotient = actual intelligence/ intelligence expected for an individual of the same age, I would recommend Gould (1981) and Gardner (1983, 1993). I share their opinion that IQ is not a good measure of intelligence and gives a limited and distorted view of the cognitive potential of an individual. However, I tested Nico's IQ to satisfy the curiosity of those who believe in it and to make a comparison with other clinical studies. In fact some authors have analyzed the IQ in hemispherectomized patients. In one of the best test studies available Peggy Gott (1973) has detected that in a child with a right hemispherectomy performed at the age of seven the IQ was just about half the one measured before illness. In our case, five years after the surgery Nico's IQ was 109 (verbal IQ 118, performance IQ 97). Certainly it has not halved! Besides Nico's IQ is also much higher than the IQs tested by Vargha-Khadem *et al.* (1991, table 2) on five right hemispherectomized children, where the highest IQ was 85 (verbal IQ 98, performance IQ 73).

We urgently need a different approach to the brain/mind correlation if we want to explain the behavior and cognitive abilities not only of these half-brained persons but of every one of us. Whales and elephants do have larger and heavier brains than ourselves but neither speak nor write. A half-brained child, on the other hand, with less than 700 grams of active neuronal encephalic tissue can speak and write perfectly well. Where does the difference lie? Do we really need so many neurons and so many synapses to be human? Science does not know – so far – how to count the number of neurons and synapses involved in "higher" mental activities, but can give a very detailed account of "motoric" neuro circuitry as has been shown by P. S. G. Stein and others (1998). Could we dream of a similar work on "thinking" neuro circuitry in the near future? I shall try to show that a hemispherectomized child can develop a normal mind although his brain has less active neurons than a microcephalic person. The difference with the latter, of course, is that Nico's left hemisphere has a normal neural architecture.

By the way, how much is half of the 10^{12} neurons of the human cortex? This is, incidentally, a good question to test the mathematical abilities of our friends or students; many will answer 10^6. This is a typical "cognitive illusion" of the type described by Amos Tversky and Daniel Kahneman (1982), and superbly summarized by Piatelli-Palmarini (1993) when our intuition contradicts our reason. The specific difficulty in dealing with power functions is also a hindrance when we deal with changes of scale, with the different orders of magnitude in the depths of the brain. We have had, all of us, a "linear" mathematical training in school and it is not easy to switch to the "power function" mode. We must learn, for instance, that half of a very great number is still a very great number! (the answer to our former question is 5×10^{11} neurons). When we say "he is brainy" or "she has brains" (in the plural) we are perhaps experiencing a neurocognitive illusion . . . But what is an objective measurement of human brainpower? And herein lies a subsidiary hypothesis: if the human cortex is so well-endowed a tissue as to be able to accomplish the same cognitive feats with only half of its neurons, then with the help of some external computational aids, would it not be possible for the brain to attain incredible levels of competence? This is the obvious inference to be drawn from our experience of the computer as an "intellectual prosthesis" in the education of a half-brained child, as we shall see later. I think that here we are at the leading edge of our capabilities as a species in a global society.

I shall finish with a practical question. What can we do to "put more brain" into education? Until now we have thought of a child's brain as a black box. But the neurocognitive sciences have opened that box and as a result some brain mechanisms have become clear, important cognitive processes have been identified and we have even been able to simulate how neural networks develop in the process of learning. All this is very distant from the demands of common classroom practice, but things are changing rapidly in education. It is no coincidence that the opening of the brain box is synchronous with the opening up of the world. We can now establish a relation between the World Wide Web and the brain wide web (Battro, 1997). The new domain of neuroeducation should deal with this complex dual network. The development of the brain wide web inside our heads and its connection to the World Wide Web around will perhaps become the new frontier of education in the twenty-first century. It reminds me of Kant's well known phrase in the *Kritik der praktischen Vernunft* about the two things that filled his mind with ever new and increasing wonder: "der bestirnte

Himmel über mir und das moralische Gesetz in mir," the starry heavens above me and the moral law within me. In a more modest way, what fills me with wonder now is the link between the two networks, the Internet and the brain.

2 Sculpting a new brain

caro m'è il sonno, è più l'esser di sasso
mentre che il danno, e la vergogna dura
non veder, non sentir, m'è gran ventura
però non mi destar, deh, parla basso

Dear is sleep to me, but dearer still to be of stone
As long as the harm and shame endure
Not to see, not to hear, is great good fortune to me:
So do not awaken me, speak low.

Epigraph by G. B. STROZZI TO *LA NOTTE* OF MICHELANGELO
(1534) TOMB OF GIULIANO, DUCA DI NEMOURS, SON OF LORENZO
IL MAGNIFICO, FLORENCE.

Look at the classic anatomical picture in any textbook, or take a solid cast of a brain hemisphere in your hands, or even better, if you are a student of medicine, handle a real brain in the human anatomy class and divide it into two parts through the corpus callosum leaving the cerebellum, the diencephalon, and the brain stem intact. Excise one hemisphere entirely and visualize the dramatic loss of brain substance that occurs to an hemispherectomized individual. I confess that I tried to model an anatomical hemispherectomy in clay but it was too difficult for me. My failure as a sculptor forced me to look elsewhere. I knew that the new technology of virtual reality (VR) was performing miracles in the field of virtual surgery, but it was inaccessible to me. The team of neuroscientists at the Kent Ridge Digital Labs (KRDL) of Singapore came to my rescue. They became interested in this case and at my request they kindly simulated on their *Dextroscope* the functional right hemispherectomy performed five years ago on Nico's brain, following the operative protocols of that surgery. I would like to acknowledge this technological prowess as a significant token of scientific solidarity from the Antipodes and I am deeply moved and grateful for their generous contribution.

Virtual surgery belongs to what is called *Computer Aided Surgery*. To quote W. L. Nowinski (1997) "the stereo virtual image of the brain is seen reflected in a mirror, allowing the user to reach into the virtual spaces. Physical and virtual spaces correspond, so that physical tools can manipulate virtual objects in a coordinated hand-eye manner". That means that

> the user's left hand controls the entire displayed complex containing the actual patient's data, an individualized 3D atlas, and a stereotatic frame fixed to the patient's head. This complex can be turned and placed as one does an object held in the hand. The right hand performs detailed manipulation using 3D widgets to interact with the surgical planning tools and the actual patient's data. For example, the user can set the frame, pull out any cerebral structure for a closer look, or manipulate the stereotatic probe. All the interactions follow the principle of 'reach in for the object of interest and press the switch on the stylus to interact with it'. Whenever the stylus tip enters the volume of influence surrounding an object, the object signals interaction readiness by a color change or other highlighting.

A new kind of medicine and psychology is emerging. In the near future this digital interface will help us to analyze not only the anatomy but also the function of the living brain, in a virtual reality setting. It is impossible to describe the feeling of having a virtual brain in one's own hands with all the possibilities for planning surgery or studying anatomy and even neuropsychology!

A VR simulation of the functional brain surgery is reproduced in figure 2.1 and is quite impressive. The virtual surgery shows that some frontal and parieto-occipital brain tissue remained intact, but during Nico's actual hemispherectomy these pieces were completely disconnected from the central nervous system and now they are no longer functional nor can they be re-activated.

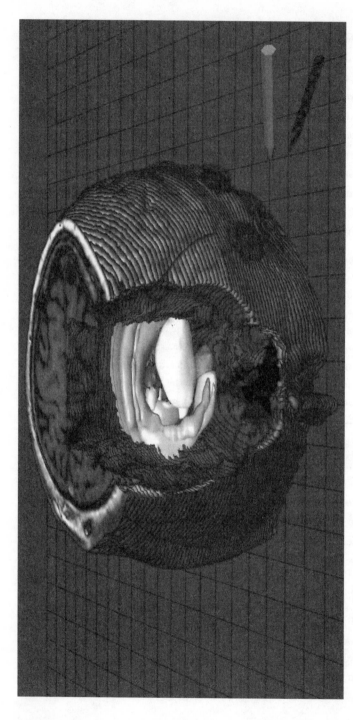

Figure 2.1 Virtual hemispherectomy. Three-dimensional view of a functional right hemispherectomy, simulated by Drs. Ralf Kockro and Yeo Tseng Tsai on virtual reality. The surgeons have reproduced the procedure performed five years before on Nico's real brain. The basal ganglia are three-dimensional reconstructions of the digitalised Talairach–Tournoux Brain Atlas, co-registered with a standard MRI of a healthy brain (courtesy of the Kent Ridge Digital Labs KRDL, Singapore).

And last but not least, thanks to the new technology of virtual reality we can now share the experience of a powerful training tool for neuroeducation and a theoretical platform for philosophical reflection. I can even imagine a new way of looking at our own brains, after an MRI performed on ourselves, though not necessarily with Hamlet's grief as he holds Yorick's skull, "alas poor Yorick! I knew him, Horatio – a fellow of infinite jest, of most excellent fancy . . ."(Hamlet Act V Scene I). Now we can hold our own brain in our hands and still fancy! But there is a paradox in the way we analyze ourselves, namely that of being at once the observer and the observed, especially when dealing with actual brains. I agree with the mathematician Alain Connes (Changeux and Connes, 1992) that "in order to avoid the paradox of intro-spection we must introduce a hierarchy between analyzed brains (of type o) and analyzing brains (of type 1)." Stanislas Dehaene (1997) in a functional MRI study of his own brain during an arithmetic task has given us a good example of this. The virtual workbench will thus provide a new interface for "neuro introspection" so that one day not only my anatomical brain but also my functional virtual brain can be analyzed. Then perhaps new kinds of thinking skills will develop, so that whenever I manipulate my type o (virtual) brain on the VR workbench I will engage my type 1 (real) brain in a new kind of epistemological subject/object interaction. This now seems to be pure science fiction but I can imagine, in the near future, the impact of "virtual brain reality" upon neurocognition and neuroeducation.

Our simulation of brain sculpting as virtual surgeons might be useful also as a metaphor when comparing our images with that of a broken computer. It is obvious that chopping a PC or a Cray supercomputer in two is a rather costly and uninteresting action. A half-brain might work as a full-brain, a half-computer cannot. Modern hardware in no way corresponds to the architecture of the living brain. Only when the gap between computer hard-ware and brain architecture is bridged will machines behave like living organs. Perhaps that day is not very distant. Both computer scientists and neurocognitivists are very much concerned now with the "minimal architec-ture" needed to perform a specific mental function. Even the idea of "lesion-ing a network" has become operational. This notion may be traced back to John von Neumann and involves a very technical computational question, but a good summary related to neuropsychology has been given recently by

Plaut (1995). Plaut gives a connectionist and dynamical approach to the problem:

> the connectionist framework should be viewed as a particularly privileged lens through which to explore and rethink development in terms of minimal architectural representability and/or computational predispositions.

What is really striking is the amazing brainpower that is left in humans who have undergone hemispherectomy – another reason not to trust those analogies between the brain and machines that have recently become so popular.

We can now analyze some facts about brain measurement that will help us to understand the quantitative consequences of hemispherectomy. The mean adult brain weight for men is about 1400 grams and for women 1200 grams. At birth the infant brain weighs circa 800 grams and will grow until early adulthood. It seems also that this growth is not as smooth as we had once believed but proceeds in stages. Also, when the brain reaches its maximum weight it starts to decrease and between age 30 and 80 a loss of 100 grams can be detected. At the same time, it is interesting to note that the surface area of the cortex and the weight of the brain are highly correlated. The implication is that convolutedness (the multiple folding of the cortex) and brain size are equivalent measures. This is most interesting because the functional relation of area to volume involves a parameter related to shape. Some authors consider the increase of convolutedness as an evolutionary solution to the problem of keeping the increasing amount of brain tissue inside the limits of the cranial volume. There is a whole province of neurological study dedicated to the measurement of the brain, but different authors give different figures for the calculation of the numbers of neurons, cortex surface, and brain volume.[1]

Table 2.1 provides a (mnemonic) schema of the order of the magnitudes involved (the figures are rough estimates), and also proposes a new terminology.

Hemispherectomy or hemidecortication roughly halves most of the number of components, but as I mentioned previously half of a very large number is still a very large number! It is in this sense that "half a brain is enough" because if we measure brainpower quantitatively, by a neuron or

Table 2.1   *Brain measurements (a power function scale)*

1 K = 1 Kilo	= 10^3	Synapses per neuron,	Kilosynapse
1 M = 1 Mega	= 10^6	Neocortical columns,	Megacolumn
1 G = 1 Giga	= 10^9	Neocortical neurons,	Giganeuron
1 T = 1 Tera	= 10^{12}	Total number of neurons,	Teraneuron
1 P = 1 Peta	= 10^{15}	Total number of synapses,	Petasynapse

synapse count alone, the amount of components that remains is still enormous. But a purely quantitative evaluation is clearly insufficient, we need a qualitative analysis as well. A hemispherectomized child may have an active brain which weighs only some 700 grams, the weight of a microencephalic brain! But these individuals are certainly not oligrophenic, on the contrary, they can perform superbly in several domains, as in the case we are discussing. This is a great mystery because these children do not behave as if they had a "small" brain at all! Many of the questions that will arise from our investigation relate to problems such as this. We are prone to providing linear solutions to non-linear problems. But this intuitive bias is dangerous. We need careful metric and dimensional analysis to deal with questions concerning half-brained cases.

In the particular case we are now discussing, Nico underwent neurosurgery at the age of three-years-and-seven-months when the average brain weighs approximately 1100 grams. Around 300 grams of brain tissue was anatomically removed, but the functional surgery has disconnected a corresponding amount of matter from the central nervous system. According to the old clinical classification, a male brain under 1000 grams in weight should be considered microencephalic. But certainly removing a whole hemisphere does not produce a microencephalic mentally retarded person! Incidentally, it is worth noting that some microencephalic individuals may show some surprising mental capacities. Donaldson (1896) refers to the case of a microencephalic woman, with a stature of 1.32 metres, who "sang and spoke readily" with a brain weighing only 289 grams at the time of her death (age forty-one)! Some recent studies have shown more striking results, as in the case of trilingual hyperlexia in a microencephalic girl (Lebrun et al, 1988). These and other extreme cases demonstrate the need for a better definition of human brain-power. It is also interesting to compare the development of the brain from childhood to adulthood in our species *Homo sapiens sapiens* with fossil brains (Saban,1995). For example the *Homo paleojavanicus* had a brain capacity of 1000 ml (similar to a present day one year-old child), while *Homo habilis* had only 700 ml (similar to a baby of age forty days). The comparison of weight is only made here because of our search for a better understanding of what brainpower means. It is obvious that brainpower cannot be identified with a neuron count. As we shall see in Chapter 3 the fundamental aspect is "neural efficiency."

Nico's congenital left hemiplegia and the onset of severe epileptic seizures in the right hemisphere at the end of his first year, coupled with the right hemispherectomy performed at three-years-and-seven-months, have made it possible for a radical re-organization of the brain to take place, something which may even have started at birth. In a neurophysiological sense Nico had been forced anyway to develop a new brain, a new hemisphere, in his first three years of life. Many questions arise, for example, what kind of meta-bolic requirements ensue as a consequence of hemispherectomy? It is said that the brain accounts for approximately 2 per cent of total body weight but needs 20 per cent of body-at-rest energy! How much energy does an active half-brain need? Does the remaining cortex activate new areas in order to accomplish the specific processing of those functions that were embodied in the removed cortex? Will some extra energy be required to compensate for the loss of the other hemisphere? These are important questions that will demand a careful design in future neurocognitive studies of a half-brain.

To begin with, brain growth is non-linear. It seems to develop by definite steps, in "fits and starts," at different rates in time and space. For instance, H. T. Epstein (1974, 1978, 1979) was able to show a biennial increment in human head circumference. He was perhaps the first to put forward the bold propo-sition of a co-ordinated link between these brain stages and Piaget's cognitive stages. Epstein coined the term "phrenoblysis" to describe the brain spurts during growth and its correlation to mental stages: "human brain weight and head circumference manifest four growth stages at about 3–10 months, 2–4, 6–8, 10–12 and 14–16 years." He reached the conclusion that "since DNA synthesis in the brain ceases around one and a half years, the last stages must be expressed mainly in elongation and branching of axons and dendrites, and in myelination of axons." Epstein also disseminated the highly controversial idea that many educational programs have failed because they focused on ages four to six, during a span of minimal brain growth. That the brain size grows in fits and starts is now widely accepted and was confirmed by different authors (Lampl and Emde, 1983, Lampl *et al.*,1992).

Of course, the measurement of head circumference is a very insufficient record of brain growth and can only be related to gross anatomical development (human brain weight is proportional to the cube of the head circumference). What is needed, as Robert W. Thatcher (1994) remarked, is to understand the functional neurophysiological changes at the microanatomical level during brain growth: axonal sprouting, synaptogenesis, myelination, expansion of existing synaptic terminals, pruning of synaptic connections, presynaptic changes in the amount of neurotransmitters, etc. A summary of the evidence concerning stages in brain growth, synaptogenesis and brain activity (EEG) is given by Kurt W. Fischer and Samuel P. Rose (1994). Coincidentally, Thatcher also uses the metaphor of "sculpting" the brain tissue. The cyclic brain growth spurts,

> may reflect a convergence process that narrows the disparity between structure and function by slowly *sculpting* and shaping the brain's microanatomy to meet the eventual demands and requirements of the adult world. According to this notion, an individual's gross anatomical structure is established early in development, and the postnatal iterative *sculpting process* is used to fine-tune anatomical structure to meet the needs of diverse and unpredictable environments. (my emphasis, p. 257)

Also,

> although the number of neurons decreases with age, the number of synapses per neuron does not necessarily decrease. This is because increased skull volume and decreased neuron number result in decreased packing density. However, decreased packing density is directly related to dendritic length. Since dendritic length is directly related to dendritic surface area, there is more space for synaptogenesis as neuron number declines. (p. 261–2)

Other scientists have studied this important issue too: Goldman-Rakic, 1987; Greenough, 1986; Hanlon, 1991; Hudspeth and Pribram, 1990, 1991; Rabinowicz, 1979.

Imperfect as they are, the current non-invasive technologies are constantly expanding our knowledge of how the brain and the mind grow together. Recent experiments provide some evidence of a stage-like growth of *both* brain and mind. Since Piaget's time and the Geneva school, several revisions of the notion of mental stage have been made. The notion of brain stages is more recent and it too will need further clarification and confirmation. The problem is how to relate the two stage-like phenomena. These considerations are vital to the study of a half-brained child. We can only infer some of these internal neural changes from his overt behavior. The idea of stage-like brain growth is founded experimentally on the data obtained from the new technologies in neurology, especially from the computerized electroencephalographic records in longitudinal studies and children's brain images. There is still a clear need to correlate brain growth and cognitive development. Later I shall discuss some intriguing results of the "brain-mind coupling" from the viewpoint of the developmental study of a half-brained child.

Using sophisticated techniques in EEG records taken from different points on the scalp it is possible to give a measure of the phase synchrony between spatially separated generators. This cross correlation is called the EEG coherence and represents the shared activity or coupling between neocortical neurons. Any increase in coherence reveals a corresponding increase in connectivity among neurons. Thatcher has discovered that "growth spurts" of cortical connectivity can be found during at least the first sixteen years of life. These spurts are measured by peaks in velocity in the coherent EEG records. What is interesting is that the growth spurts in connectivity are cyclic. He observed three cycles: I (from 1½ to 5 years), II (from 5 to 10 years), III (from 10 to 14 years).

The passage to the next cycle is always marked by phase transitions (or discontinuities) in the EEG records. This last fact provides a strong argument for a stage-like development in neuronal connectivity. Moreover, and this is central to our study of half-brained children, the growth spurts take place in different predominant locations during brain development. For instance, Thatcher observed six left and two right-hemisphere growth spurts between ages 1½ and 2½ years, as the cycle moves from predominantly left to bilateral. The nesting of micro-cycles and sub-cycles in every major cycle can also be shown. According to the author the developmental sequence of the cortical neuronal networks of the left hemisphere "is from short-distance differentiation to long-distance integration," while "the right hemisphere begins with a long-distance integration of distributed subsystems and then progresses to short-distance differentiated or specialized subsystems" (p. 253). In his view, during neural development the right hemisphere integrates differentiation (short to long-distance neural connections) and the right one differentiates integration (long to short-distance). This can be related to an anterior-posterior anatomical *expansion* (left hemisphere) and *contraction* (right hemisphere) in the cortical system's connections. But also, approximately every four years, there is a lateral to medial *rotation*. The sequence "begins at left lateral cortex, then intrahemispherically expands to left dorso-medial cortex, then projects through the corpus callosum to the right dorsomedial cortex, and finally intrahemispherically contracts in the right cortex" (Thatcher, 1994, p. 244). The whole developmental picture of the growing brain can be synthesized as "two-year growth spurt cycles in the strength of intrahemispheric couplings, which are nested within four-year interhemispheric rotations."

If this is the growing neural pattern of connections in the normal brain, what will happen in the case of a half-brained child? The standard model should be challenged against the new situation, where the interhemispheric rotation of neuron connectivity is anatomically impossible (as is also the case in split brain patients). In our case Nico has undergone a right hemispherectomy in the middle of his first cycle (three years) at which time it is possible a bilateral growth spurt in neural connectivity was taking place. Nico, who at the time of this writing is eight years old, cannot iterate the spurt of bilateral connections, as a bilateral-brained child is expected to do. What sort of new connections are being established in his half-brain? We do not know. We should design an equivalent EEG experiment to test the neuronal growth in half-brained children on a rigorous physiological basis and look for differences from the standard pattern.

And what about the problem of cognitive stages and their relation to brain stages? Fischer has given an overall view of the correlated sequences of both.[2]

There also seem to be cyclic iteration of front-to-back power EEG spurts in the growing brain, which follow the construction of the cognitive developmental steps, called levels. Each level of skills presupposes the emergence of a new kind of neural network. Levels belong to larger cycles, called *tiers* by Fischer. He affirms that at the beginning of every tier (emergence of actions, representations or abstractions) a spurt of neuronal activity is detected by the power EEG technique in the frontal areas, followed by an occipital-parietal, then a temporal and finally by a central spurt, and restart again in the following tier with the same sequence. Like stages in Piagetian theory Fischer's tiers represent different levels of dynamic cognitive stability. This is an intriguing and important question to analyze.

The new assumption is that the frontal cortex plays a key role in the reorganization of all cognitive abilities at each developmental stage or tier. It would be interesting to discover whether the left half-brain will also show similar front-to-back spurt cycles in neural activity, irrespective of the neural effect of the right hemispherectomy. The fact is, as will be described in Chapter 4, that Nico displays no delay in the acquisition of mental skills, as assessed by the classic Piagetian tasks. To sum up, we are dealing with new and fascinating discoveries in the intimacies of the relation between postnatal cortical development and child cognition. The panorama is open to further research, in particular when a hemisphere has been anatomically or functionally removed. The new technologies might open an operational window to identify the way the half-brain reorganizes its neuronal circuitry and our quest for a measurement of brainpower should continue through the description of the many parameters involved in brain growth. It has been shown that purely quantitative analysis at the gross anatomical level (loss of neuronal tissue, etc.) is clearly insufficient. We need a detailed account of the architecture of the new neuronal networks in the half-brain. It is the hidden quality of this design that makes our brain powerful and efficient.

same time with the localizability of damage and the non-localizability of complex psychological functions! *A fortiori*, focused lesion analysis cannot be applied in hemispherectomy, where an entire galaxy of neuronal components has completely disappeared. Again, it is clear we need a positive approach in order to understand cases in which lesion analysis is inappropriate. Bach y Rita (1990), for example, describes how the brain self-generates "rehabilitation programs" to overcome damage. The alternative I am now proposing may be called "compensatory analysis."

Faraneh Vargha-Khadem and Charles E. Polkey (1992) produced a very thorough review spanning twenty years of publications on the cognitive effects of hemispherectomy or hemidecortication as a treatment for severe epilepsy. The results were encouraging. Not only did most children survive the drastic removal of a hemisphere but some of them, as in Nico's case, have shown such a remarkable readaptation in every activity that we cannot consider them to be living with a "damaged brain." They live with an intact brain. An intact half-brain. They enjoy life, friends and family, learning and playing. Their partial motoric (hemiplegia) and visual (hemianopia) loss makes them no more disabled than others who suffer from a peripheral neuromuscular trauma or disease. Nowhere is the coexistence of "broken brains and normal minds," as described by S. M. Kosslyn and M. van Kleeck (1990), more clearly expressed than in hemispherectomized persons. It is interesting to quote their main points:

1 Functional components cannot be identified with symptoms.
2 Functional components need not be neatly implemented within the brain.
3 It is difficult to determine the function-implementation mapping.
4 Behavior is determined by multiple components.
5 Quantitative deficits can produce qualitative effects.
6 Localization of the lesion does not necessarily localize the damage.
7 Descriptions of deficits are theory related.

The conclusion is that these children or youngsters should not be treated as having damaged brains! Parents, educators and physicians need to focus primarily on their motor rehabilitation (and on speech and linguistic training in cases where the left dominant hemisphere has been removed). In some cases, such as Nico, the degree of motor recovery can be astonishing. Immediately

3   Compensatory analysis

*Dos o tres veces había reconstruido un día entero;
no había dudado nunca, pero cada reconstrucción
había requerido un día entero.*

*Two or three times I had reconstructed an entire day;
I had never hesitated, but each reconstruction took me an entire day.*
JORGE LUIS BORGES, *FUNES THE MEMORIOUS. 1944*

In this book we are discussing a very extreme case of brain damage, hemispherectomy, an extensive lesion provoked by neurosurgery as a means to cure a disease, such as intractable epilepsy. I shall argue, however, that hemispherectomy is more than a neurological lesion. In my opinion it amounts to rebuilding a new brain, to inducing a new neuronal architecture in the remaining hemisphere following the removal of its counterpart. This half hemisphere is functionally transformed into a whole brain again. If half a brain is enough then half a brain amounts to a whole brain. Concepts such as brain efficiency, compensatory process, equipotentiality, self-reorganization, vicarious functioning, neural plasticity, prostheses, and the like, need to be carefully analyzed in this new context. Much of the actual progress in the neurosciences is based on "lesion analysis," a methodology employed by most experimentalists and clinicians but perhaps never so well described as by Hanna and Antonio Damasio (1989). Their definitions merit a detailed discussion if we want to sort out the identity of hemispherectomy. We will begin with lesion analysis first in order to get to compensatory analysis later.

First,

> *Lesion method is the establishment of a correlation between a circumscribed region of damaged brain and changes in some aspect of an experimentally controlled behavioral performance.*

Hemispherectomy is the anatomical or functional removal of a complete hemisphere. As such, it is not a circumscribed region of damaged brain that will be correlated to certain behavioral performance but an intact hemisphere, a healthy half-brain, that might be experimentally tested. Thus, the lesion method cannot be applied, *stricto sensu*, in this case, because the active half-brain is, at face value, undamaged. The follow-up of some hemispherectomized patients can show functional troubles in the remaining hemisphere, as shown, for example, by EEG records (Smith *et al.*, 1991; Müller *et al.* 1991). In Nico's case, no spikes or abnormal waves were detected in his left hemisphere, before or after surgery. The pre- and post-surgery MRIs also have shown a normal left hemisphere. We can infer that he has a healthy half-brain. Hemispherectomy amounts to a huge loss of components of the central nervous system, and a complete topological and topographical change in their connectivity. In this sense, as I said, it is the equivalent of sculpting a new brain.

Second,

> *Given a preexisting theory about the operation of the normal brain and how it would mediate the performance of an experimental task, the lesion (the area of brain damage) can be seen as a probe to test the validation of the theories, that is, a means to decide if the account of brain organization and operation provided by a given model is or not falsifiable.*

This point is crucial, the method must be related to a theory. Philosophers of science have explored this relation in great detail. And, as often happens, they came out with incompatible theories about the validation of models. The theory invoked here is that a model cannot be proved as such, it can only be falsified or not (Popper, 1965). But how a model should be subjected to an empirical test in order to be validated is still a controversial theoretical issue. Philosophers and methodologists do not often agree about the required criteria but scientists continue to develop models and tests without much debate.

It seems that a standard agreement has already been reached in the prac science, theories of science notwithstanding.

This way of thinking is a common methodological assumption amo entists today and operates in most cases. But, in my opinion, it is dif apply in the case of hemispherectomy. In fact there is not, as we have area of brain damage to be tested. The damaged hemisphere h removed. The empirical behavioral testing should be performed on half-brain. This is not a point of detail but a central one. For insta will show, it is extremely difficult to predict a specific cognitive de the lack of an entire hemisphere. Accurate inferences and detaile tions, by contrast, are common in lesion analysis, in instances brain damage area is correctly identified. There are hundreds of p books on the neuropsychology of brain-damaged patients (incl brains), but few surveys of the developmental, cognitive, percep or social aspects of hemispherectomized individuals. Compare massive neurosurgical intervention in such cases the deficits or behavior in these patients are relatively minor. For these cases alternative methodology to lesion analysis, a positive approach brain.

Third,

> *As a consequence, the smaller the lesion probe capa discriminatory effects . . . the more the lesion metho contribute.*

Current neuropsychological assessment can evaluate very and lesion analysis should provide the corresponding ratic measurement (Lezak, 1995). In extreme cases, lesion ana applied to the experimental microscopical removal of a neurons, as minute as a minicolumn of the cortex, for e extreme minimal level of damage the theory can certainly be rigorous scientific test of falsifiability. However, this is not a clinical neurology where brain damage often implies the de lions of neurons and connections. As Damasio (1994, p "neuropsychology is not, or should not be, about finding t tion' for a 'symptom' or 'syndrome'." In many cases, we m

after neurosurgery he could not walk at all. Now, five years later, he runs and plays, with only a slight limp. He gained motor control via the ipsilateral connections of the left brain. His left arm movements are limited, but when forced to use his left hand he can often reach the intended target. Sometimes, for instance, he uses a finger of his left hand in order to hold down a key to capitalize a letter on the computer. The most remarkable outcome, of course, is that, so far, no significant cognitive or affective disorder has been identified in this half-brained child. The question is: how will his potential develop in the future? The scientific literature is not very specific about long-term quality of life after hemispherectomy. We also lack sound statistical information about the cognitive abilities of a half-brained child beyond elementary school. Will Nico succeed in finishing high school and entering university? There is always a possibility that at some point in his psychological evolution there will be a breakdown and a failure at school as a consequence of a developmental arrest. We should be cautious and well-prepared to monitor his efforts to meet clearly defined objectives in his formal education. As I write this book many people are helping Nico to become a good student. At present there appear to be no obstacles to a successful completion of his elementary years, but it is difficult to make predictions.

In a sense we are leaving the neurological and educational domains now and moving into philosophy. Perhaps one of the most interesting examples of the philosophical use of brain-lesion analysis was given by Maurice Merleau-Ponty in his two books *La structure du comportement* (1942) and *La phénoménologie de la perception* (1944). He made an intensive study of the findings of the German neurologist and Gestalt psychologist Kurt Goldstein (1934) which relate mainly to the perceptive and cognitive effects of brain wounds. Some fifty years later the American thinkers Patricia Smith Churchland (1986) and Paul M. Churchland (1996) have developed a new discipline called "neurophilosophy" in which lesion analysis still plays a major role.[1] With the exception of the few pages Popper and Eccles (1977) have dedicated to the cognitive effects of hemispherectomy, no consistent reflection on half-brained patients has, to my knowledge, yet been undertaken by a philosopher. But, as I have said, we cannot explain the consequences of the removal of a complete brain hemisphere by classical lesion analysis. We would need a

different kind of analysis not only in neuropsychology but also in neurophilosophy. I believe compensatory analysis could be a valid alternative.

The main requirements are as follows: first to focus on what is left, not on
what has been removed, and second, to describe how the half hemisphere
develops into a full and healthy mind. The first aspect relates to the fact that
the remaining hemisphere is providing "substitutes" for many functions previously performed by the removed one, as we shall see. The second is an invi-
tation for compensatory analysis to be performed over the entire life span of
those individuals who have undergone hemispherectomy.

We expect these children will show a normal psychological development
but also, in a very precise sense, the half-brained child can be considered an
"exceptional child." He certainly develops a "high-ability-halfbrain": a half-
brain that performs as a whole brain! This fact does not always imply giftedness, but does not exclude it either. The eventual spurt in neuronal efficiency
in half-brained individuals can be tested by compensatory analysis. For
example, we may compare the biopsychological cluster in the gifted
described by Norman Geshwind and Albert Galaburda (1987) with the conditions exhibited by Nico.[2]

The Geshwind-Galaburda Syndrome (GGS) correlates five traits of very
different type to giftedness: superior spatial skills, non right-handedness,
bilateral cortical representation of language, language related problems and
immune system disorders. This interesting mix of talents and handicaps, of
gifts and deficits, shape a new kind of pathology: "the pathology of superiority" as it was called by Geschwind. An explanation for GGS is an altered
brain organization due to an increase of testosterone in the fetal brain. Nico,
a right hemispherectomized child, is the perfect mirror image of GGS: he performs poorly in some spatial tasks such as drawing, he is right-handed, he has
a definite left cortical representation of language and no language related
problems or immune system disorders. The altered brain organization in this
"inverse GGS" case is primarily the result of two causes: first, of the congenital left hemiplegia and the functional effect of an early devastating epilepsy
when the right cortex seizures interfered with his left non-epileptic cortex
and, second, the anatomical effect of neurosurgery at age three. The combi-
nation of these successive injuries "forced" the left cortex to assume the functions of both hemispheres. It is in this sense that we may speak of

overcompensation. It is known, from animal research, that when some cerebral tissue is removed (in monkeys) the other brain compensates for the loss by an increase in growth (Goldman-Rakic and Rakic, 1984). Also, an intact left brain is necessary (in mice) in order to develop an intact immune system (Renouz, 1988; Cardinali *et al.*, 1997). Both conditions seem to be fulfilled in Nico's case with the development of a new neural circuitry in the left brain. This might represent a kind of compensatory growth for the removal of the right brain and raises the important question of neural space and "neural crowding" in the remaining hemisphere.

If the left hemisphere can develop the skills of a whole brain, it follows that it has enhanced its efficiency. In fact, recent investigations of the way in which the human cortex consumes energy in the performance of different skills can provide valuable information. Non-invasive brain imaging techniques can be used to measure the consumption of glucose, the brain's fundamental source of energy, during clearly defined mental tasks. It seems, for example, that the high-ability brains of gifted persons are more efficient. That is to say they consume less glucose at the same time as performing better than the control ones (Haier *et al.* 1992; Posner and Raichle, 1994). Similar experiments should be conducted at some point on half-brained individuals in order to rigorously test their neuronal efficiency. This notion will help us to enrich and qualify the concept of brainpower.

In our subject the so-called right hemisphere skills – mathematics, visual arts, and music – have migrated to the left hemisphere. We must stress that Nico has no particular gift whatsoever in these skills but neither is he deficient in them. At school he performs like any other child of his age in arithmetic and music. Only his draftsmanship and his handwriting are poor for his age, but this does not involve a real loss of his cognitive spatial performance. Perhaps Nico has only shifted from an "analog" to a "digital" style in these abilities. In fact he can make good graphic designs with the help of a computer, and is mastering written language with the aid of a word processor. In the verbal domain, a left brain skill, Nico, performs well above average. A normal linguistic performance might be expected in his case but not as advanced as it actually seems to be. However, we cannot exclude the possibility that Nico might have had an exceptional verbal brain before surgery. It is impossible to test this assumption now but the point is that there is no reason why a half-brained child should not also be a gifted child! As the number of half-brained children increases it is possible to imagine a longitudinal study of a cohort of children with high-ability half-brains. This program could take its inspiration from Lewis Terman's famous "study of genius", which started in 1921, but without its theoretical limitations (Terman and Oden, 1959). Nobody would deny the importance of a study that keeps track of hundreds of bright children (Terman's subjects were called the "termites") over the course of their entire life. Some of these children are now in their eighties! What will the life of a half-brained person be like at that age? Perhaps we might see the development of a new kind of giftedness in such high-ability half-brains. We need to keep track of them. They could turn out to be the termites of the twenty-first century!

We can now discuss some definitions for compensatory analysis. I would like to suggest the following three, in the hope that they might at least be of some use as heuristic tools:

First,

> *Compensatory analysis is the establishment of a correlation between the part and the whole, and in our case in particular, between the half-brain and the whole brain, by controlled experiments.*

Thus the properties of a half-brain should be correlated to the properties of a whole brain, i.e. a double half-brain. This is not an easy task either for the experimental neurosciences or in terms of methodology.[3] The compensatory analysis of the new circuitry in the half-brain will confront the strict logical problems of the extension of sets of neurons, with the inclusion of one subset in a set, and so on.

Second,

> *Given a preexisting theory about the operation of the whole normal brain and how it would mediate the performance of an experimental task, the half-brain can be seen as a probe to test the validation of the theories, that is, a means to decide if the account of brain organization and operation provided by a given model is or not falsifiable.*

Instead of a damaged area we have here an intact brain hemisphere which acts as a probe to test the general theories of the mind and the brain. Until now these theories have benefited enormously from lesion analysis but not so much from the study of hemispherectomy. In a sense, compensatory analysis sets out to validate a system from within the system, the whole from the part.

Let me give an example of compensatory analysis in vision. Because of his brain surgery Nico suffers a complete left hemianopia. He cannot see the left part of his visual field. He is constrained to move his head in order to focus on a visual target. The visual images that are formed in the left nasal and right temporal retinas cannot be transmitted because of the incomplete section of the corresponding pathways. In a normal brain the signals of the right hemi-retinas travel through the optic nerve, optic tract, and optic radiations to the right primary visual cortex along the calcarine sulcus (the striate cortex or Brodman area 17 or V1) of the occipital lobe of the right hemisphere. Because of the hemispherectomy, Nico's right neocortical pathway (geniculate-cortical pathway) has been disconnected and his stereoscopic vision depends, exclusively, on his left occipital cortex. This is why the testing of the central processing of three-dimensional images can give us some vital information about hemispheric compensation. As far as I know there is no such information in the current literature on hemispherectomy. A good opportunity to apply compensatory analysis.

The interesting thing is that we can now perform a kind of "visual psycho-anatomy" with a half-brained child, and analyze his central process of vision for stereopsia. In fact three-dimensional vision is supported by retinal disparity (the left and right visual fields do not overlap completely). Stereograms are artificially produced with two slightly different views of the same object, which can be fused with the stereoscope. The fusion is produced at a central level, some four synapses at least past the receptors (rods and cones) of the retina: bipolar and ganglionar retina cells, lateral geniculate neurons (LGN), and cortical neurons of the primary visual cortex. There are no synaptic junctions of the right and left visual pathways at the LGN. The first contact is made at the visual cortex. Thus the information coming from the two retinas is not combined until the first cortical stage V1 and is reprocessed at the extrastriate cortex V2 (area 18). The main point is that the central nervous system can combine any stimulation pair and extract the information that is hidden to the peripheral process. Bela Julesz (1971) called this particular type

Figure 3.1   Random-dot stereogram. When monocularly viewed it appears as an aggregate of dots. When stereoscopically fused a diamond is perceived in the center hovering above the random-dot background. The corresponding anaglyph should be viewed with red and green eye filters (from Julesz, B., *Foundations of cyclopean perception*, Chicago University Press, 1971 © 1971 Bell Telephone Laboratories Inc.)

of central processing "cyclopean vision." He discovered a clever method of by-passing the peripheral process by means of random-dot stereograms which provide no familiar perceptual cues to the retina. When viewed monocularly, the random-dot patterns of figure 3.1 will provide the reader with an example of this. These patterns "do not tell" the retinas anything in particular. We can discern no shape in them. But when viewed through a stereoscope (or when green and red filters are used to view the corresponding anaglyphs) the reader should see a diamond shape that pops out from the background. This striking phenomenon is particular to the cyclopean vision of higher mammals, even a human infant can react to and stare at an elevated shape such as a central square hovering over the random-dot background. The use of random-dot patterns in this kind of experimental procedure introduces the observer directly into the visual cortex. This is a compelling reason to study the cyclopean vision of a half-brained child, particularly because stereopsis has been reported to be a right hemisphere-dominant process (Carmon and Bechtold, 1973).

In an experiment which Nico found most amusing, I tested him with the colored anaglyph versions of five random-dot black and white stereograms provided in Julesz' text, inviting him to use a viewer with red and green filters, one color over each eye. In most individuals, though not all, the cyclopean view produces a strong depth effect which can be reversed by reversing the filters. This is a good test to control the subject's description of the visual three-dimensional image. Where is the "cyclopean-eye" located in a half-brained child? It is certainly not a geometrical construct midway between the two eyes. Compensatory analysis should help us to understand whether or not one visual area alone would suffice to produce a cyclopean visual image. From what we knew about Nico's abilities we were able to predict a perfect compensation. And this turned out to be the case. Nico performed with ease in all the tested visual tasks. He reported the appearance of a diamond, a square, a letter T, a saddle and a spiral shape, in the corresponding random-dot anaglyphs using the red-green goggles. His cyclopean eye is clearly supported by his left visual cortex alone! This fact corresponds to the prediction from the compensatory model of a "whole cyclopean brain" inside his left hemisphere.

Third,

> As a consequence of that, the greater the loss of nervous tissue capable of creating compensatory effects in the remaining part of the brain the more the compensatory method will have to contribute.

In other words, what is the minimum brain architecture capable of acting as a sustainable probe in compensatory analysis? This is, I admit, a purely speculative problem in the context of contemporary neurology, but it could turn out to be a practical issue in the future, when an artificial neural prosthesis could be connected to the brain. Perhaps the best exploration of this question is in a book of science fiction written by one of the founding fathers of Artificial Intelligence, Marvin Minsky, and the novelist, H. Harrison (1993). We can imagine, for instance a brain/computer physical interface that would create a new dual – organic/artificial – nervous system. At present, however, the minimum sustainable neural organization for compensatory analysis is the half-brain.

4　First schooling

the gods don't hand out their gifts at once,
nor build and brains and flowing speech to all

THE ODYSSEY, BOOK 8, 167–8
HOMER (TRANS. R. FAGLE, 1997)

My friend Nico is a normal child. Only his brain images remind us of his brain condition. This is a kind of well-kept secret inside his skull. If Nico is invited to a party where nobody knows about his medical history, he is welcomed as an attractive child with a slight limp and some restriction of movement in his left arm and hand. It is impossible to infer from his overt behavior what has actually happened to his brain. But the computer magnetic resonance images are there to remind us of his neurosurgery. And he knows that too. He does not actually know the technical details but if asked he will say he underwent brain surgery when he was small. He regularly undergoes medical tests, EEGs and the like, and he took anticonvulsive drugs for some three years following surgery, but no longer needs them. He is certainly a healthy, charming boy.

When I first met Nico he was five years old and I did not know much about the extent of the surgery performed two years earlier. His parents came to ask for precise advice on education and computing for him. I was not consulted as a physician but as a pedagogue. I asked, however, for a detailed account of the neurosurgery protocols and some recent images of his brain. I immediately started to work with him at a computer in order to evaluate his visual

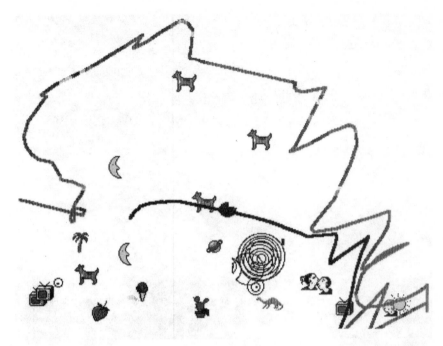

Figure 4.1   First computer graphic at age five. Nico learned to move and copy small
images of people, animals, plants, and other objects on the monitor.
He also used the mouse to draw lines and curves on the screen. The
result was a fascinating computer art composition.

and motor capabilities when using the mouse and the keyboard. Nico was
very friendly towards my assistant and me and we were quite impressed to see
this hemiplegic boy trying so hard to operate the computer. He displayed no
visual neglect on the screen and in a few minutes he was able to click and drag
the mouse with ease.

I observed that he loved using the computer more than the usual toys he
was offered. He was hyperactive throughout the whole session. He was eager
to play with icons, letters and colors but was so excited that my assistant and
I had difficulty in following an organized program on the computer. He liked
changing tools, erasing, exploring. In the six sessions that followed, however,
we succeeded in making Nico carry out some simple Piagetian tasks, such as
seriation and classification on the computer screen. He was able to perform
one-to-one visual correspondences with the icons but could not seriate

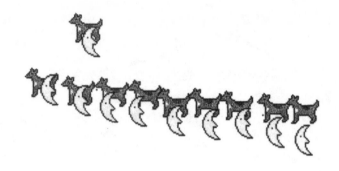

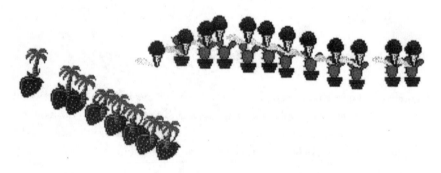

Figure 4.2   One-to-one visual correspondence on the screen at age five. The computer task was to copy and paste a collection of small images and to put one above the other (dog – moon, strawberry – palm tree, ice cream – cactus).

consistently. His verbal comments about his computer work were incredibly articulate, witty and humorous, and showed a remarkably rich vocabulary. It was not until the end of this evaluation that I received the corresponding neurological records and brain images. I could not believe my eyes! Nico had had a complete functional right hemispherectomy yet was performing on the computer like any normal child of his age.

My recommendation to the family was to start a normal education with the aid of computer tools. Accordingly I went to talk to the headmaster of a traditional school, with a good reputation, willing to accept Nico in kinder-garten. I had the good fortune to know the headmaster of that institution quite well. In fact I had been working for a number of years as a consultant on 'digital education' in several teaching and learning activities, and the school was already prepared to accept the technological (computer and communica-tions) challenge to make the necessary digital shift to help Nico. Taking care not to over-simplify the problem, I explained how important it would be for Nico, his family and the school, to take up this educational challenge. We did not have the slightest idea how to teach a half-brained child. He agreed to have a go. The first year at school was a kind of day-by-day experiment. The teachers were informed about the case and everybody took pains to find new ways to help this charming hemiplegic child in his daily activities. His hemi-spherectomy was not mentioned again. What Nico needed was a pleasant environment in which to grow up. And so it was.

In the first months at kindergarten he was often tired, but he was given plenty of time and space to relax on a mattress or take a nap. He was then taking a mild anticonvulsive medication. His companions were very kind to him and the adults grew more and more confident as his teachers. The educa-tion of this exceptional child was becoming a natural and common task for all. Nico was very happy at school. It is an excellent school with more than one thousand students of both sexes, at primary and secondary levels, advanced computer and communications equipment, large buildings, exten-sive gardens and open fields. It is a private school with a solid reputation earned from decades of teaching, not a special school for handicapped children.

After kindergarten Nico was accepted in first grade without any problem, but we were concerned about whether he could manage the stress of formal learning. He did very well. He also started to attend classes in English as a foreign language in the afternoons, in which he is now obtaining the highest grades! He did not exempt himself from any school activity. Furthermore, he had a good attendance record throughout the year. Only gymnastics and sports were specially tailored for him, taking into account his motor disabil-ities, with an emphasis on his long-term rehabilitation. I recommended giving Nico a laptop computer, and this was done. His computer became his copybook. He also had the use of his father's PC at home and another one in his class, but Nico was the first pupil at that school to carry a laptop computer around. In fact a portable computer is a perfect tool for students of all ages, but for some reason adults are reluctant to give them one. For Nico it was not only an innovation but the perfect companion, and more than that, the computer became his "information prosthesis," to use Seymour Papert's phrase (1978). And now, thanks to his example, the whole class is moving forward. Pupils, teachers and parents are now learning to use email. And the remarkable fact is that Nico is leading the transformation! There is a moral lesson here. The more I work with disabled people the more I learn that they are teachers. "The one that you are supposed to carry will really carry you," as Paul Claudel (1957) said in his *Prière pour les paralysés*: celui que tu crois porter, c'est lui réellement qui te portera.

There is a myth about handwriting being the 'educationally correct' way to acquire literary skills. But in Nico's case, there was no justification for not allowing him to use a typewriter from the outset. He had too much difficulty in holding down a sheet of paper or a copybook with his left, disabled, hand. As I have mentioned, Nico is still behind for his age in drawing skills, and he has real difficulty in forming the letters of the alphabet and numbers with his right hand. I shall return to this important point later, when we discuss the differences between 'analog' and 'digital' perceptual and cognitive abilities in a half-brained child. To sum up, with the aid of a computer Nico learned to write and was able to keep up with the normal pace of his class. Nico mastered the basics of spelling and grammar at the same age as most normal children do. He loved writing long sentences on the computer and seeing them printed in Spanish, his mother tongue, or even in English.

The following are some typical texts produced by Nico at different ages with the aid of a computer. It is amazing how well he uses the word processor to write, correct, delete and print. The computer is his favorite tool to copy a text, compose a description, take down dictation or write a letter.

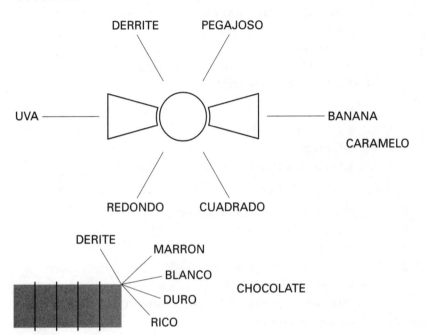

DIA   MIERCOES21

GOLOSINAS

DERRITE   PEGAJOSO

UVA   BANANA

                                    CARAMELO

REDONDO   CUADRADO

DERITE

MARRON

BLANCO

DURO   CHOCOLATE

RICO

Figure 4.3   A computer task at age six: To write the attributes of a candy (raisin and banana) "melts, sticky, round" and a chocolate: "melts, brown, white, hard, good."

age 5:
Copy
LEON
MAMA

age 6:
(a) Description
DIA MIERCOLES 10
HIDROPONIA
FORMA DE CULTIVAR PLANTAS QUE NO NECESITA TIERRA
NECESITA AGUA I SALES MINERALES.

EXPERIMNTAMMS:
1—ELEGIMOS LOS MATERIALES
2— PONGO LAS SEMIYAS
3—RIEGO CON MUHA AGUA
Day, wensday 10
Hydroponics
Way to cultivate plants that don't need earth
Need water and mineral salts.

We experiment:
1. select the materials
2. I put the seeds
3. I sprinkle with a lot of water

b) Assignment:
PARA TENER UNA LINDA SONRISA DEBEMOS
SPILLARNOS LOS DIENTES
IRA DENTISTA
NO MORDERCOSAS DURAS
COMER POCASGLOSINAS
COMER CARNE FRUTAS LECHE VERDURAS PESCADO
LAVARNOSCON FLUOR

To have a nice smile we need to:
brush our teeth
go to the dentist
do not bite hard things
eat few candies
eat meat, fruits, milk, vegetables and fish
wash with fluoride

age 7:
a) Dictation
DIA VIERNES 2 DE MAYO
DICTADO
LA CASA DE I TIA QUE DA EN OLIVOS
MI MAMA COSINO UNA RICATORTA.
EN EL JARDIN FESTEJARON EL DIA DE LOS ABUELOS
MI BANDERABLCO SELESTE

Day Friday 2 May
Dictation
The house of my aunt is in Olivos
My mother baked a good pie.
In kindergarten they celebrated grandparents' day
My flag is white and blue

b) Description
DESCRIPCION SOBRE EL HORNERO.
SU COLA ES ROJISA.
CUANDO TIENE UNA CRIA ABANDONAN SU NIDO Y HACEN OTRO.
EL HORNERO CANTA PARA ENAMORARSE
MIDE 20 CM.EL NIDO PARECE UNA PELOTA DE FUTBOL.
Description of a bird (hornero).
Its tail is reddish.
When they have a chick they leave their nest and make another.
The homero sings for love
It measures 20 cm. The nest looks like a soccer ball.

c) Letter
QUERIDO ANTNIO
TE SPLICO QUE SE ME ESTA CALLENDO UN DIENTE.
APRENDI QUE EL HUESO MAS LARGO ES EL FEMUR.
TE PIDO QUE VGAS A VISTARME AL SALON PERO UN RATO LARGO.
UN BESO
NICO
Dear Antonio
I tell you that I am loosing a tooth.
I learned that the longest bone is the femur.
I ask you to come to visit me in the classroom but for a longer time.
a kiss
Nico

age 8:
Nico's first email
HOLA ANTONIO SOY NICO. FLOPI ESTA BAILANDO LAURA NO ESTA EN ITALIANO.

TE QUIERO MUCHO. NICO.

Hi Antonio! I am Nico. Flopi is dancing "Laura is not here", (a song) in Italian.

I love you much. Nico.

The process of handwriting is cumbersome for all children, whereas type-writing is always easy. Pressing a key on the computer is much simpler than holding a pen and making a mark on a paper. Even now, after two years of handwriting practice Nico has consistent difficulty in mastering this particu-lar skill. He still inverts Ns and Ss, writes capital letters too large, and mis-places letters or words on the horizontal lines, etc. His poor handwriting is in marked contrast with his skill on a word processor. Stressing the absolute necessity of a computer from the outset to help Nico in his learning process was the right choice. (This issue will lead us to a discussion about word pro-cessing and the brain, confronting texts and hypertexts.)

And what happened with regard to his reading abilities? We know that the cortex that writes is not the cortex that reads. We also know, from lesion analysis that agraphia and alexia are separate neurological disorders (Gibson and Levi, 1985, Gray and Kavanagh, 1985). We can say that with his intact left hemisphere Nico should be cognitively well-equipped to read, but what about his defective left visual field? Nico has a left hemianopia because the functional hemispherectomy has severed all the neural paths that project the hemi-right retinas to his disconnected right visual cortex. How then does he manage to read, and read so well? This is an open question that will require further investigation. Nico has a very particular way of moving his head in order to focus his central field of vision. We can also expect to find an atypical pattern in his saccadic eye movements during reading.[1] But the fact remains that he reads and enjoys reading very much. And how does Nico get on in arithmetic? He is good at that too. Nico is a good learner and enjoys numbers. The same goes for music. He loves to sing and has memorized many melodies and songs. Nico is an average child in his class in most tasks, at the top of his class in verbal (oral and writing) skills, towards the bottom in drawing. He could be described as a typical "verbalizing" and not a "visualiz-ing" child, in the terms used by Howard Gardner (1982).

But schooling is much more than a learning program. It is a learning human environment in which social and emotional skills are required to develop an identity. Nico is a child who suffered from intractable epilepsy, which began in his second year of life. It was by all accounts a devastating condition with constant seizures, loss of consciousness, fear and medical treatment which culminated in critical brain surgery performed abroad, a long way from home. Nico remains a highly sensitive child, overprotected at times by his family and friends. He has a younger brother and a sister who attend the same school and there is a clear rivalry between the siblings. What could be expected at school of a child with such a background? Some emotional and affective imbalance perhaps, due to the complete removal of his right limbic system, amygdala and hypocampus? There is also some evidence of a right dominance for emotions (Gainotti, 1972, Heilman *et al.*, 1983, Borod, 1992). But, the expected symptoms did not appear. On the contrary, Nico behaves like any emotionally balanced child of his age. Nor have we detected a specific "attention deficit disorder," which is so common at this age. He is friendly towards everyone, young or old; he has a remarkable sense of humor; he is very affectionate and popular; he loves and is loved.

Nico has undergone several Piagetian cognitive developmental tests in a longitudinal study which we expect to continue (Piaget and Inhelder, 1963). We have not yet found any sign of impairment or deviation in his cognitive abilities. On the contrary, he has shown a normal development of all the abilities we have been testing. For instance, we observed that at the age of five-years-and-eleven-months he reached the stage of the conservation of quantity for the 1–1 correspondence between icons using the computer as a tool. According to the Piaget-Inhelder scales, 50 per cent of children of his age also reach this stage. The conservation of substance was tested in the standard way with two small, identical clay balls, A and B. B is then transformed into a sausage B'. The "conserver" child affirms that A and B' still have the same amount of clay. The arguments offered by Nico related to the conservation of 'identity' under transformation. When tested at the age of six-years-and-four-months, he had reached a full conservation of substance, a stage only reached by 16 per cent of children according to the same Genevan scales. However, at the age of six-years-and-four-months he was a non-conserver for quantity of liquid. The conservation of liquid was tested using a simplified technique: two glasses of identical shape and volume (A, B) contain the same amount of water; then the water of one glass (A) is poured into a larger but shallower glass (A'). The question is whether there is the same amount of water in B and A'. Nico gave non-conservatory answers using the same kind of argument as that reported in 40 per cent of children of the same age: "A' has less water because it's lower." When tested seven months later, however, he had attained full conservation. In the test of seriation of rods of increasing length we made use of the computer to draw lines of different color and length, in order to improve his motivation. At the age of five-years-and-eleven-months we obtained a typical stage I response but by the age of seven he had reached stage III seriation with a correct intercalation of (solid) rods. At the age of six-years-and-six-months he was tested in logical thinking (class inclusion) with a bunch of ten flowers B, consisting of eight roses A and two daisies A'. He was able to quantify the two subclasses within the whole class of all flowers B (A+A'=B). Only 13 per cent of children of his age quantify class inclusion. To sum up, we detected no significant developmental problems, according to these standard Piaget–Inhelder tests.

The conflict between what could be termed the 'analog' and the 'digital' cognitive skills in mental development is an interesting point. The technical terms analog and digital are essential to the computer sciences but are not so widely used in psychology. However, they can help us to have a better understanding of the plasticity of the human brain subject to hemispherectomy. As we have seen, Nico has poor drawing skills. Drawing is a highly analog activity in that it is mostly continuous and smooth at the motoric–gestural level. However, Nico is very skilful on a computer with a mouse, the equivalent of a pencil. Moving a pencil or a mouse are both analog activities, but the mouse has the "click option," and this can make a significant digital shift in our spatial abilities. Computer graphic software is a good instrument with which to evaluate the "digital aspect" of the spatial skills of an individual of any age. In the case of a right hemispherectomized child this digital shift amounts to forging a new way of representing space with the left hemisphere. In fact Nico has an astonishing ability to move in hypertextual space, where buttons and icons may open new windows, change colors and shapes, produce sounds, create drawings, and letters, etc. As I have mentioned, his "analog drawings" and his representation of space and objects in two dimensions are some two or three years behind his age, but in the organization of his digital cyberspace he is well ahead of his class! Other interesting results have been

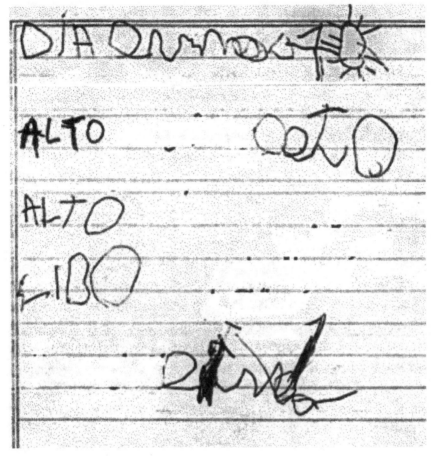

Figure 4.4   Handwriting at age seven. Nico shows poor writing skills with a pen while he manages to produce a good text with a computer.

obtained with the Raven Progressive Matrices test. The problem consists of completing geometric matrices of increasing difficulty. Nico performed at an advanced level, solving thirty-five out of the thirty-six figures tested (percentile 95). This is a remarkable result for a right-hemispherectomized child who would be expected to perform poorly in non-verbal thinking tasks.

The difference between perception and the representation of space is also a good theme to investigate with a half-brained child. Piaget, Inhelder and Szeminska (1947, 1948, 1961, 1966) studied this cognitive problem in depth. For instance, they were able to show that the perception of the horizontal evolves independently from its representation. A classic test is to request a drawing of the horizontal level of a liquid in a tilted glass. Most children aged six draw a line perpendicular to the sides of the glass, yet Nico drew an oblique (though not quite horizontal) line, and his results were the most advanced of his whole class! This is quite striking in view of the fact that, in the first place, Nico shows poor drawing skills and, in the second place, most researchers agree that the right hemisphere is responsible for processing geometric tasks (Franco and Sperry, 1977). But in all the tests I have so far conducted, I have been unable to find any specific deficit or impairment in spatial or geometric thinking. His drawings of trees planted on the side of a hill are also correct, all pointing upwards instead of fanning out as most children of his class still draw them. I shall discuss below the clever way in which Nico wrote his first Logo program to draw a geometric figure. Perhaps we are reaching here a point of bifurcation, where drawing skills and geometric concepts split in a half-brained child. In Nico's case the latter seem to be more highly developed.

It might be useful now to summarize our findings using Howard Gardner's framework of multiple intelligences (MI). Gardner (1999) has identified at least eight different intellectual capacities: interpersonal, intrapersonal, linguistic, logical-mathematical, spatial, musical, naturalist, and bodily-kinesthetic. I shall attempt to sketch Nico's mental profile using the MI framework. Our pupil excels in interpersonal relations. He is a leader in many situations involving verbal interaction. It is interesting to see how he behaves in a social situation, for example. I first noted this when I invited him to visit my home with his family. I have a nice garden but rather than going out to play he preferred to stay with the adults, asking questions about everything and participating in our conversation. If I ask him to do a drawing he will take the time to give somebody else a pencil so they can do one too. He does not like to work in isolation but prefers to share his activities. It is also interesting to record his group behavior at school. We videotaped him during some psychological tests at school. When we invited some of his classmates to do a Piagetian test with him he explained the task to the others; for instance, the best way to classify a collection of objects, etc. Nico has many friends of both sexes. They help him in many ways, especially when he is having difficulty in reaching an object or doing some hard manual task. During his second year at

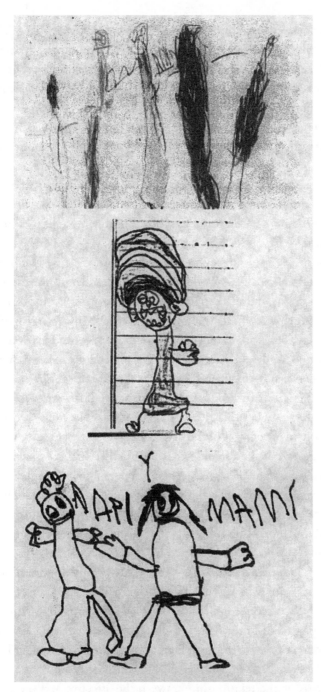

Figure 4.5   Three typical drawings at ages six, seven and eight. Nico shows
poor drawing skills, but he is now making significant progress.

school he underwent reparatory surgery in his disabled left leg. When he returned to school in a wheelchair everyone was vying for the right to push him along which he enjoyed immensely. When he first started at school he used to wander incessantly and spend a lot of time flitting from one activity to another, dreaming up new things to do or interrupting the others while they worked in class. Now this hyperactive behavior has disappeared and he has become less restless (or lazier?). He frequently waits for his companions to finish their work before starting his own. He often asks for help or says he is tired and refuses to work. Perhaps he is beginning to suffer from the stress of school competition. When he fails to finish his work in time he has to work late at home with his mother's help. But he loves school and what he is doing there. Although to some extent his performance at school is cyclical, when properly tested outside the constraints of the classroom, his cognitive competence is growing steadily. Nico always works on his computer but he also attempts to work conventionally and this can lead to problems. We know for certain that the computer empowers his learning skills, but there is always a risk of a progressive décalage between his inner cognitive capabilities and his overt school production. And we all know how difficult it is for a school to keep a harmonious balance between both dimensions of learning. It is for this reason that we are aware of the need to introduce the class as a whole to the sphere of new computer technology in order that they may all share in Nico's work. Once again we return to the parable of the weakest individual in a group stimulating his stronger peers to make a significant change in their collective habits.

Interestingly enough, Nico gives us many opportunities to explore in some detail how aware he is of his own identity as a half-brained child. His intrapersonal intelligence manifests itself in some insightful comments about himself and it can be both moving and amusing, to observe his use of his brain disability to justify an instance of laziness at school. One day, for example, he told his teacher that he was tired and could not finish his work because, "as you know," he said, "they operated on my brain." We shall closely follow Nico's conceptual and emotional constructions on the specific subject of being a half-brained person. We know that there are many ways of becoming aware of an action. Jean Piaget has written a celebrated book on that topic, *La Prise de conscience* (1974), in which he explored the developmental process of the relationship between the affective and the cognitive unconscious. The philosopher Daniel C. Dennett in *Consciousness Explained* (1991) discusses split brain experiments which demonstrate the new ways which patients find to do the same tricks they used prior to surgery. Maybe we should re-define consciousness in the context of one hemisphere alone doing all the exploration.

Nico's linguistic intelligence is remarkable. He began speaking quite fluently before the age of two and lost no linguistic ability at all following surgery. Nico's verbal performance is now above average. This is not simply because he has scored 118 in verbal IQ (which is in any case a somewhat controversial measure of linguistic ability), but because of the richness of his vocabulary and syntax. A conversation with him is always interesting. He can give a lively account of any particular event, be it a holiday trip, a video or a sporting activity. He has a pleasant voice and speaks with great self-possession. It is a pleasure to hold a conversation with him. I have suggested stimulating his linguistic skills by learning easy poems and dramatizations, which he seems to enjoy very much. It is also interesting to note his joy at learning a second language. In the afternoons he attends English classes at school, in which he attains a high level of success, and has a collection of English songs at home which he loves and knows by heart. The extent of the so-called "neuronal crowding effect" in his left brain needs further exploration. So many compensatory functions and still enough 'room' to incorporate a second language and maybe others as well!

His written language skills, on the other hand, seem to need extra space – a kind of external memory. As I have said, his laptop serves him as an "intellectual prosthesis." It would be extremely difficult, if not impossible, for Nico to remain at school without this empowering instrument. And lately an innovation is bringing about a significant change: email is now transforming his life. We have prepared an interface to enable him to select any of his digital penpals with a single click, and I am on his list. What does it mean to an eight-year-old half-brained child to be connected to the Web? Nico has a close extended family, some of whose members live abroad, and they usually communicate through the Internet. His classmates and teachers are also beginning to use email; Nico is now in contact with some of them. As Papert (1997) says, he belongs to a "connected family"! This development has far-reaching implications for his linguistic intelligence. For instance, it stresses the pragmatic dimension of language. Although syntax and semantics are formally taught at school, "how to do things with words" in the pragmatic use of language – is somehow a mystery. Consider how many letters or memos are written in a year by a pupil in the third grade and what they convey! In general, whilst the requirements of the school curriculum may be satisfied, the children's real interests are not. Email on the other hand is an enormously powerful pragmatic tool for all of us, children and adults alike. I must confess how proud I was of Nico when, using my computer, he sent his first message to a dear colleague of mine at Harvard! When I first met Nico such a feat would have been difficult to imagine . . . The enormous impact on Nico's life of the new computational technology is still a source of constant wonder to everybody. Email is one of the bridges that technology is building around us. This is only a beginning, but I can predict a qualitative leap forward when the whole class interacts with Nico on a daily basis.

Nico loves music. A recent gift from me was a beautiful radio I brought back from Singapore. I know he is enjoying listening to it (I always try to make him participate in my travels – next time we should be in contact by email). I have a piano at home and the first time he came he asked my permission to play. I tried to teach him a short tune with his right hand and he was eager to learn. Every time he visits me he asks to go to the piano and he enjoys playing with an electronic musical keyboard at home. He needs some help with an instrument like this, but fortunately, nowadays, digital synthesizers can supply the left-hand accompaniment. At school he is learning to play some simple percussion instruments and he enjoys singing, whether solo or in a choir. The development of a musical intelligence in a right hemispherectomized child is certainly a challenge for neuroeducation. It may be of interest to note that some authors have detected a difficulty in locating sounds which are contralateral to the ablated hemisphere. For instance, a right hemispherectomized sixteen-year-old girl was subjected to a precise auditory test, the results of which were worse for moving sounds than for stationary sounds (Poirier et al,1994). Of course, this would not seem to present a major obstacle to a serious musical education.

It is in the act of drawing that we see Nico's principal cognitive deficit, but I have no proof that his visual-spatial intelligence is impaired. This raises a very interesting point of discussion. Many authors have linked the right hemisphere to spatial processing. As I have already mentioned Nico's spatial sense was "forced" into his left hemisphere, first by the epileptic and disabled right hemisphere and subsequently by surgery. Furthermore, his left visual field is impaired. It is quite remarkable how he compensates for this major visual deficit by means of eye and head movements in most situations. As a consequence of the hemianopia his reading ability is somewhat diminished. He reads well but cannot follow the written lines easily, or at least not at the same speed as his classmates. It is a well-known fact that the saccadic eye movements in the process of reading are very precise, that they improve in efficiency with practice and undergo specific changes when there are visual or brain lesions. I fully expect that with continuous exercise his eye-scanning pattern will improve and that new reading methods will develop with age and practice. This expectation is supported by the impressive example of Nico's ability to process three-dimensional cyclopean images with his left visual cortex against all the odds.

Nico is perfectly well oriented in space and time. With the exception of drawing I have so far been unable to find a single specific cognitive impairment produced by the right hemispherectomy. I have tested some aspects of his precocious spatial ability by means of the representation of the horizontal level of a liquid in a tilted cup. And now, at the age of eight, he has revealed full operatory spatial thinking in some Piagetian tasks: the construction of a projective line using the alignment of solid objects between two marks on a table. And if we shift to the circumscribed space of the computer screen, Nico's spatial performance is outstanding. He drags the mouse with ease and moves the small cursor with great precision and without hesitation. I shall discuss below how well he manages to program the translations and rotations of a turtle on the screen using Logo computer language. But his drawing by hand is still well behind his spatial cognition. We are currently offering him a wide variety of possibilities and techniques for improving his drawing abilities.

Logical mathematical intelligence has been widely identified as a predominantly left brain activity. But studies on left hemispherectomized children show that under certain circumstances the right hemisphere can, to a large extent, compensate for the loss of the dominant hemisphere. Correspondingly, the development of logic in a right hemispherectomized child such as

Nico should not be a problem. In fact I could show that his logical thinking follows the normal developmental pattern. This is important because for Piaget the concept of number is the operative synthesis of classification and seriation. But how does the transition from an "unschooled mind," as defined by Howard Gardner, to scholastic learning take place in a half-brained child? How is Nico learning arithmetic at school? He has told me several times that he greatly enjoys arithmetic and he is very proud of his good grades. But although he appears to have no specific difficulty in the subject areas of elementary arithmetic and geometry and has no difficulty in keeping up with the rest of the class, he shows no particular talent for mathematics. His main gift is for language. Nico is also developing as a budding naturalist. He is collecting all sorts of specimens and he told me he wanted to start a small museum at home. In this task he is collaborating with his younger brother.

Finally, let us attempt to describe Nico's bodily-kinesthetic intelligence. A right hemispherectomy produces a left hemiplegia and left hemianopia. These are Nico's principal disabilities and they are in striking contrast to his cognitive and emotional capacities which are predominantly intact. His motoric handicaps are now the main focus of concern to family and teachers alike who try to provide him with the best physical rehabilitation available. From a neurological point of view he has some voluntary control of the axial and proximal set of muscles in his left limbs. These control the elbow, shoulder, hip and knee via the ventromedial corticospinal (ipsilateral) tract which represents one tenth of the pyramidal fibers coming from the left motor and premotor cortex. Nico's motoric rehabilitation depends on this secondary bundle of ipsilateral connections (Müller *et al.*, 1991). Thus, his remaining left hemisphere has the potential to control the proximal movements on both sides of his body. But the lack of contralateral motor connections from the right cortex via the lateral corticospinal tract disrupts the voluntary control of the distal muscles, especially of his left hand and fingers.

When I first met Nico he was a very slim, delicate boy. Now he has grown and is capable of some physical activities which were impossible a few years ago. For instance, he can now go up and down a long staircase at school several times a day without assistance. He also achieves a reasonable level of outdoor activity at school despite his hemiplegia. He successfully underwent orthopedic surgery in his left foot at the age of seven and his gait is now improving. His father is a sportsman and has first-hand knowledge of the beneficial effects of physical training. He became his son's coach in more senses than one. Nico likes swimming and has recently discovered tennis. But for obvious motoric reasons, I imagine, he intensely dislikes soccer – he even refused to watch the national team playing in the World Cup in France on TV! Careful motoric rehabilitation will certainly help to enhance the bodily-kinesthetic intelligence of a half-brained child. To sum up, as expected, Nico shows the superior language skills of a left brained child. But we now also have a more coherent view of the large number of compensatory effects which take place following hemispherectomy, particularly in many spatial tasks. The discussion of these and other, as yet undiscovered, developmental facts may in future help us to obtain a clearer understanding of the underlying neuro-psychological dynamic.

5   The cortical shift

The Brain – is wider than the Sky –
For – put them side by side –
The one the other will contain
With ease – and You – beside

EMILY DICKINSON, 1862

We are now ready to take a further theoretical step. In the place of standard lesion analysis we have proposed compensatory analysis as a means of dealing with hemispherectomized individuals. We have also collected some psychogenetic data from the first school years of a half-brained child with a normal mental development. I shall now deal with the notion of "cortical shift": the substitution of one brain area by another. This relates both to compensatory analysis and to education. In our case Nico has developed a new left brain in the sense that it performs many of the neural functions currently attributed to the right hemisphere. A cortical shift probably began at birth (or even before) because of his congenital left hemiplegia, then went a stage further at the early onset of his epileptic seizures and was firmly established following surgery. But there are other – artificial – means capable of producing a more specific kind of cortical shift. These are the computerized tools of today, which may act as genuine intellectual prostheses.

I want to show that with the help of computers it is possible to activate new brain areas and perform new cognitive tasks. For instance, when we use a word processor we organize new writing schemes which differ from those used in handwriting or typewriting. We have set up a new cognitive space on the screen which supercedes the cumbersome task of writing with paper, ink, rubber, tape, glue, scissors, and stamps, and enables us to edit, print, save, and mail with ease. It is not simply the substitution of the old instruments by the computer keyboard that makes such a difference but the use of different cognitive strategies. It is not a motor change but a mental change. And different writing strategies entail the activation of different cortical areas too. Thus, just as a hemispherectomy forces a massive cortical shift, so may computers also elicit a more (limited) cortical shift. As we shall see, both the natural and the artificial cortical shifts gently merge in the education process of a half-brained child. But we must now take a detour to explain the impact of computers on cognitive development in general before discussing their role in the education of a hemispherectomized child.

Digital processors are machines that have changed the way we interact with the environment, with other people, and with ourselves. In particular they have changed the way we interact with our brains. The essential unit is a triad which comprises the person P, the machine M, and the environment E: {P, E, M}. The environment is either exogenous or endogenous. The brain belongs to the latter. The triad is internally connected by the symmetrical relations PE, EM, MP. These represent the three possible functional interfaces between: the person and the environment (eg. a pencil), the environment and the machine (eg. a sensor) the machine and the person (eg. a word processor). Each triad can be connected to many other triads. The fundamental external connections are of three kinds: person to person PP, machine to machine MM, environment to environment EE. These three (not always symmetrical) external connections are of different physical natures. A face to face communication is a PP relation (audio-visual-gestual). The network between computers on the Internet is an example of an MM connection. The interaction of photons and the retina is a case of an asymmetrical functional relation EE between the endogenous environment of the brain (the neuronal layer of rods and cones) and the exogenous illuminated environment. The network between a pair of triads is reflected in a prism which allows a multiplicity of functional connections via different pathways and nodes. Let us suppose a teacher is on the telephone to her principal (PMMP). At the same time she makes a gesture with her hand to motion a student to come in (PP) whilst monitoring the printout

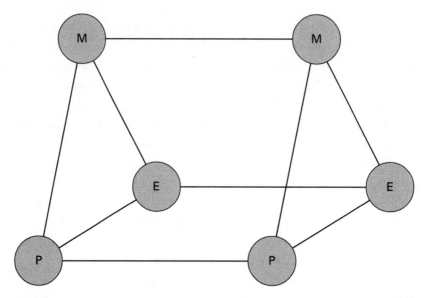

Figure 5.1   The connecting prism between Persons (P), Machines (M), and Environments (E).

of the memo (PME) she is sending via the local area network to the printer in the library (PMME). The connecting prism is activated here in four parallel ways emanating from the same source (P: the teacher).

This simple image may be useful in understanding the different relations between the components of our world, made up of artificial and natural things. The computer is "the machine of machines," the paradigm of the artificial, as Herbert A. Simon (1981) has brilliantly pointed out. The brain is, of all known natural objects, the most complex. Computers are now MM interconnected through the World Wide Web (WWW) by the millions. Brains have an inner-connectivity EE greater by many orders of magnitude than the WWW. I propose to call this EE network the "brain wide web (bww)." The idea of EE and MM as two interconnected fields might also help to give a wider view of our amazing capacity for connection as human beings. In the present case, the half-brain remains connected to both the natural and the artificial world.

In fact, Nico uses a computer to write, a digital machine that has changed his life and his experience of learning. As we have seen, instead of being handicapped by his poor handwriting, the word processor enables him to develop his writing skills with ease. In the prism of connectivity he is following a longer path PME instead of taking the handwriting shortcut PE. He is better trained to use the machine than most children of his age. Furthermore, he has no trouble sending an email via the Internet at the highest level of distance interaction PMMP! This is the essence of the notion of an information prosthesis – it enhances human connectivity. The consequences of digital networking for the individual and society are considerable, particularly when the user is a disabled person. A half-brained child on the Internet is not a dream now, but when I talked about this possibility three years ago it sounded too good to be true!

And this is not all. With the computer's help his half-brain is capable of empowering its own inner-connectivity by making use of new cortical areas. This relates to the cortical shift in the brain which a computer can accomplish. Here we must take another detour to explore briefly the new field of information prosthetics before returning to the analysis of the artificial cortical shift in the half-brained child. The idea of using the computer as a cognitive tool for the disabled was introduced by Seymour Papert at MIT in 1978. He coined the expression "information prosthetics" at a time when few could imagine any possible humanitarian use for computers. This technological and sociological breakthrough opened up new ways of improving the quality of life of physically and mentally handicapped persons (Valente, 1983). Inspired by these remarkable models I myself became totally involved in the new field (Battro, 1986; Battro and Denham, 1989). I would now like to define "intellectual prostheses" as a subset of information prostheses in general. Indeed the latter category also includes "physical prostheses" (cochlear implants for the deaf, computerized limb stimulation for quadriplegics, banks of electrodes in the visual cortex for the blind, etc.). The intellectual prosthesis by contrast, does not imply any physical or direct contact between the nervous system and the computer. It is a purely functional prosthesis not a physical one. However, we can expect both "intellectual" and "physical" information prostheses to interact in the future in ways we can scarcely imagine today. To sum up: intellectual prostheses are computational devices which interface with human cognitive activities such as speaking, writing, reading, drawing, etc. In particular, they can "open" new cognitive pathways in the brain, produce a significant amplification of cognitive performance and the functional substitution of impaired cortical areas (Battro, 1994).

The notion of the cortical shift came to me when I was attempting to teach a quadriplegic architect how to use a computer. He was diagnosed as having multiple sclerosis at the height of a brilliant career and was forced to stop working. Our aim was to design an interface to communicate with the machine. The only choice was a voice recognition device, following the connection path PME. The learning process began with the vocal control of a "screen turtle" using the Logo computer language, initially with simple instructions (such as Forward and Right, Papert, 1980). He learned how to draw two dimensional pictures. Then, with the help of more powerful three-dimensional Logo instructions (such as Pitch, Roll and Veer), he began to draw elementary figures in space. The graphic results of three-dimensional Logo can be very beautiful and it gave him the ability to experiment with different scales and perspectives (Reggini, 1985). Having mastered voice-controlled Logo the architect embarked on a systematic training with voice-controlled CAD (Computer Aided Design). After several months of intensive practice he developed amazing vocal skills for drawing and was able to make a successful return to his profession as an architect. By means of a digital network link with his office he was able to send the layouts and plans from his home, where he worked. The connectivity was established via a complex series of interfaces, PMME. The end result was the printout of the architectural project at a remote printer (Battro, 1994).

From a neurocognitive point of view it is interesting to analyze the difference between the practice of prosthetic drawing using speech recognition devices, and common hand-drawing. The difference between the two situations is in the topology of the cognitive pathways activated in the brain. It is known that many cortical areas are involved in saying a word. Even the cerebellum is active during a simple speech utterance (Posner and Reichl, 1994). Other cortical areas however are involved when moving the hand, as in the act of drawing or typing. Used as an intellectual prosthesis, the computer functions as a switch to pass from one modality (hand-drawing) to the other (speech-drawing).

Drawing by hand is a typical analog skill. Speech-drawing, by contrast, is a digital one in the sense that spoken sentences are chains of discrete elements such as words, syllables or phonemes. When drawing by hand the cognitive pathways must be kept open to continuous motor control. This is not necessary when the artist is drawing vocally with the aid of a computer because of the digital nature of speech. For example, it is difficult, if not impossible, for an aphasic artist to make a computer drawing using only speech instructions because of the specific language impairment. Yet the analog cognitive pathway used to make a drawing by hand may remain intact. It is recognized that a right-handed draftsman can produce the same pattern as a left-handed one, i.e. it is quite impossible to distinguish between brain dominances from the quality of the drawing. Moreover, clinical practice shows that even with severe (written or spoken) language impairments, many right-handed hemiplegic aphasics can readily learn to use their left hand to draw and paint.

One thing is certain, before the arrival of computers no human mind had ever produced a drawing using speech instructions alone (although in ancient Peru, Inca architects were known as "the men who give orders aloud"). We cannot imagine Michelangelo drawing up the plans for St Peter's by giving his assistants step-by-step instructions on how to produce the layout, or painting the Sistine Chapel by shouting out "some red there" or "a line here" to his apprentices. Nowadays, however, such a feat is technically possible. A computer can make such a cortical switch possible. When a human operator uses his voice to draw he activates a new neuronal network never previously engaged in the act of drawing. This switch to a new cognitive path is the essence of every intellectual prosthesis. In other words, intellectual prostheses help the brain to perform cognitive tasks previously processed by a totally different area of the cortex. Neuronal networks can be substituted or bypassed by new cognitive paths driven by computer instructions. This fact has very important consequences in clinical practice and special education, particularly in the education of a half-brained child.

The "architect who drew with his voice" followed a learning process involving a sequence of prosthetic tools: Logo 2D, Logo 3D and finally CAD. The teaching of geometry at school also starts with two-dimensional flat figures and ends with three-dimensional volumes. This is a secular pedagogical tradition dating back to the times of Euclid, and even for Piaget, the spontaneous cognitive development of Euclidean geometry follows this two-dimensional to three-dimensional sequence (Piaget, Inhelder and Szeminska, 1948). But perhaps this sequence is not so formally ineluctable or psychologically compelling, as was thought. Computers can radically change the teaching of geometry and graphic design, and also our view of the cognitive processes involved. For instance, we are now entering the virtual reality VR era which will transform the way we look and manipulate things. The post hoc (VR) simulation of Nico's right hemispherectomy illustrated in Chapter 2 is a pertinent example of this.

Let us analyze Nico's specific difficulty with drawing by hand, his "analog" drawing using a pen, and the alternative strategy of "digital" drawing using a computer. We can compare the two cognitive processes, analog and digital, with the use of a simple but powerful computer tool such as Logo. Papert's original idea was to enable the user, usually a child, "to teach" the machine to produce a drawing (and many other things) on the computer screen. The small figure of a turtle on the screen behaves like the actual tip of an electronic pen. Nico is learning Logo at school and he likes it very much. One day I asked him to draw a bridge (a rectangular figure) using the simple instructions Forward and Right. He carefully began to explore how these two instructions moved the turtle, step by step: Forward 40, Right 90, then Forward 40 and Forward 40 again. In order to make the turtle "go down" he typed Left 90, but the turtle "turned up," a common error. He corrected the rotation by typing Right 90 and Right 90 again. This is an interesting strategy for coping with a subtle question of orientation in space. Finally he ended with a Forward 40, and the "bridge" was complete. Nico arrived at a satisfactory solution by using local on the spot corrections via the visual feedback on the screen, the "direct" mode of teaching the turtle (pen) to draw. I next tried to explore a higher cognitive process which the "procedural" mode would imply, i.e. to write a small program in abstracto, without the benefit of the visual feedback from the turtle on the screen. Nico was receptive to new things that day and he wrote a Logo procedure without hesitation:

```
To bridge
Forward 40
Left 90
Forward 40
Forward 40
Left 90
Forward 40
End
```

He repeated the numbers 40 and 90, but he switched from Right to Left, which shows that he had not simply memorized the previous sequence of instructions but was creating a new way of doing things. When he typed "bridge" a neat, correct rectangular drawing appeared on the screen. He was amused and continued to type the word "bridge" making many new drawings. The session finished at that point. Nico returned to class and I began my analysis of the cognitive process involved in this simple but highly significant procedure. I have been working with Logo and handicapped children for nearly two decades and I am still convinced that it is a remarkable educational tool. But now, in the neurocognitive era, I feel that Logo might also offer a new and simple way of identifying the cortical shift in some spatial and geometric skills. For example, as we know, Nico is unable to use a ruler and set square with his left – disabled – hand and his capacity to draw geometric figures (the connecting path PE) with his right hand is therefore greatly reduced.

The important thing is that after a brief explanation Nico was able to conceive and execute some simple Logo procedures which produced correct geometric designs. In less than ten minutes he learned to program the machine (the path PME) to produce a diagram of a rudimentary bridge. Elementary though this graphic production might be, it is a cognitive feat. First, it supposes an accurate representation of the screen space and second, a sufficient command of the computer language. Besides "turtle geometry" is an "intrinsic" geometry, the concepts of left and right only make sense "locally" without reference to the actual computer co-ordinates or to the user's own body schema. Any Logo teacher knows how difficult it is for a child to detach the concept of right and left from the corresponding parts of his body when the turtle on the screen is "pointing down," for example. How much more difficult must it be for a right hemispherectomized, hemianopic and hemiplegic child with a lopsided body scheme! Not only does Nico's left brain compensate for the geometric skills of the missing right cortex, it is also an indication of the intra cortical shift from an analog to a digital representation of geometric shapes. Programming the figures in abstracto on the computer screen implies a cognitive anticipation of the graphic results and a fair representation of the computer procedure.

One year later Nico was able to carry out some more complex programs with Logo (using microworlds, lcsi). In a couple of sessions he produced a

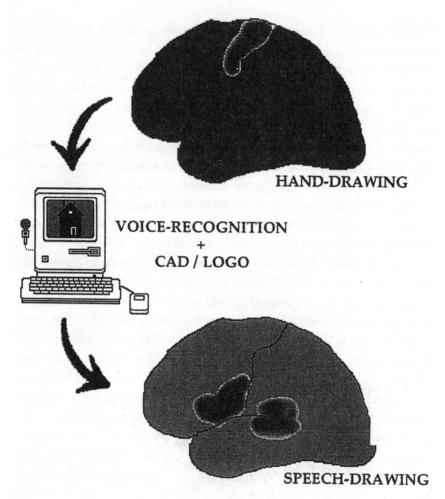

Figure 5.2   The computer can switch the brain from one cognitive mode (hand-drawing) to the other (speech-drawing).

remarkable piece of art, a frame of colored squares with his signature. This is an example of the dual property of his graphic skills. On one side he has written the instructions "to square" and "to frame" (using "repeat . . . square"), a purely digital task. On the other, he has used the mouse to draw and paint the letters of his name in the center of the picture, an analog task.

I predict that brain imaging will soon reveal the disparity of the cortical processes involved in this particular cognitive substitution of the analog by the digital language. Such a disparity has also been discovered in the cortical location of first and second natural languages (Dehaene *et al.*, 1997).

Nico enjoys using the computer. It is gratifying to see his laptop always open during class hours. This is the realization of a success story made possible by the continuous work and tireless technological efforts of a multitude of scientists and teachers round the world over the last two decades. Nowadays there is almost no sensory or motor impairment that cannot be overcome by an appropriate prosthetic device (Borden, Vanderheiden *et al.*,1994). In Nico's case any standard computer can be used because he needs no special aid to operate the keyboard, control the printer, hear the sounds or see the images on the monitor. He is also lucky to have so many computers at his disposal and, what is even more important, to be the recipient of so much good-natured support in his computer work. The principal cortical shift in his left brain, forced in the first instance by the disabled right epileptic brain and subsequently by the right hemispherectomy, is empowered by this secondary cortical shift produced by the computer which substitutes his poor handwriting and drawing. Here then we have a double cortical shift in the same half-brain: one biological – the left hemisphere taking on most of the functions of the right hemisphere, the other artificial – the computer operations which change the very nature of writing and drawing and open new cognitive pathways in the brain.

6   The double brain

What we can put on our shelves
we should not put into our brains

AUGUSTE FOREL

Rudyard Kipling (1927) wrote a poem that deserves a reading and a moment's thought, in the light of what we have been describing:

The Two Sided Man

Much I owe to the lands that grew –
More to the lives that fed –
But most to Allah who gave me two
Separate sides to my head.

Much I reflect on the Good and the True
In the faith beneath the sun
But most upon Allah who gave me two
Sides to my head, not one.

I would go without shirt or shoe
Friends tobacco or read,
Sooner than lose for a minute the two
Separate sides of my head.

The bilateral symmetry we have in common with all other human beings is unquestionably a marvelous gift. Conversely, a broken symmetry seems to disrupt the biological harmony of the whole.

The poet's eulogy of the two-sided head is in marked contrast with the reality of a half-brained person who has lost one side. It is true to say we do not give much thought to our remarkable double brained status. It requires an explicit mental effort or a poet's spark of inspiration to become conscious of it. We do not feel our brains. But how would an hemispherectomized person react to the the poem's theme? Personally I think he should be proud of his exceptional situation. A respected journalist wrote in the same vein about another eight year old right hemispherectomized child: "I can imagine Matt telling his dates ten years from now – You won't believe this, but I have half a brain –" (Swerdlow, 1995). I must confess that in the course of writing this book I became so involved in the problem of the half-brain that at times I experienced a strange mixture of awe and delight about the "wet web" inside my own skull. The terms *wet web* or *wet computer* have a deep impact on our ego; they somehow undermine our supposed robust neurobiological foundations and expose a more fluid inner state. A similar sense of fluidity came to me as a young physician after analyzing mountains of EEG records; when I closed my eyes before falling asleep I sometimes saw a disturbing sea of endless electric waves (see also the essay about the *wet mind* by Kosslyn and Koenig, 1992). The dictionary definition of awe is "a wondering reverence tinged with fear inspired by the sublime" (Webster, 1991). I kept repeating to myself that the wonder is inside our heads. And I tried to imagine what it would mean, as the poet said, to lose for a minute one side of my brain. The real wonder is that some human beings are endowed with only one side of a double brain.

The notion of a broken right-left symmetry in the brain comes from Marvin Minsky. I think it is important to quote it in full as it is insightful comment from one of the creators of the concept of artificial intelligence and relates to the consequences of a right hemispherectomy.[1]

> I do not deny that there are important predispositions for specializa-
> tion in the brain – but my guess is that these are largely optional. My
> theory: after a certain point in development, when the child has
> acquired many different resources for thinking, then (in harmony with
> what I called Papert's Principle) it becomes necessary to build higher
> level systems to manage those resources. Now, higher-level thinking
> requires deeper and more sequential operations. This is because a
> system that tries to do many things in parallel will therefore become

more fragmented – in the sense that the different activities will have to compete for limited resources of various sorts. If this is permitted then each of the parallel processes will become more stupid. It is a myth that it is good to use parallel distributed processes – because this leads not to cooperation but to mutual interference. Accordingly, as a child develops higher systems, it becomes necessary to break the right-left symmetry! *A deep intellectual process can serve only one master*! So normally, one side of the brain becomes the master at deliberate sequential planning. What happens to the other side? My conjecture: in the end, it becomes largely wasted – because it remains childish while the other side matures! This is why, in split brain adults, the (usually) right side seems more romantic, less critical, more imagic, less symbolic, etc. It is because it has been left behind, because it has less well developed managers. Now (more conjecture), the managers have simpler jobs, really, than the systems that finally do the work; they use only a small proportion of the brain. In this case there is not much loss – because it only lacks a largely redundant childish copy.

Minsky is not alone in this view about the redundant nature of the right brain. The great zoologist J. Z. Young wondered whether the right hemisphere might be "merely a vestige" and the late neurophysiologist Sir John Eccles dismissed the right hemisphere as a "mere computer" (an epithet which is in itself a vestige of the old brain/computer controversy). However, there is enough evidence of the role played by the right hemisphere in the normal and damaged brain. The point is not to deny it but to understand the way it may be substituted by the left brain.

I would now like to summarize some experiments, both old and new, involving a large team of collaborators, in the hope that they may add some neurological evidence to Minsky's theory of the agents or managers in the "society of the mind" as it relates to the half-brain. Over 1000 children and adolescents (4 to 18 years old) were tested for hand, eye and foot dominance (Battro, 1981, 1996, see note 2).

Conservation of length

Two 14 cms rods were mounted on two parallel rails and could be moved in either direction by one hand. The experiment began with the two rods A and B facing each other. The child introduced one hand through a hole in the screen which hid the rods from view and explored the length of A and B. The experimenter asked whether they were the same length; if the answer was yes one of the rods was slightly displaced to the right and the same question was repeated. The displaced rod was then returned to the first position and the same question was repeated. Finally, the other rod was displaced to the left and the experimenter asked the same question again. The answers were classified according to Piaget, Inhelder and Szeminska (1948): pre-operational children said that the displaced rod became longer, operational children affirmed the conservation of length, i.e. that both rods were the same length and that only the position had changed. The conservation of length was significantly increased ($p = 0.015$) in the RH group of children (4 to 8 years old, N=256) using the right hand. In LH children by contrast, no statistically significant difference was found between the right and the left hand groups (N=92) although a mirror inversion of the performances appeared.

Conservation of substance

The child was told to put one hand through a hole in a screen and touch two small balls of clay A and B of equal size. The experimenter asked whether A had the same amount of clay as B. The child was then invited to transform one of the balls (B) into a sausage (B'). The question was then repeated for A and B'. The answers were classified according to the criteria established by Piaget and Inhelder (1941). Conservation of substance is established when the child affirms that A = B' because while the shape may have changed, the amount of clay is unchanged, or because the objects are equal, nobody having added or subtracted a piece, etc. These answers imply concrete operations. Figure 6.1 shows the results of 152 RH (4 to 12 years old) and 80 LH (4 to 8 years old). The RH group performed significantly better with the left hand ($p = 0.0042$). There was no significant difference between hands in the LH group.

Class-inclusion

Using one hand, the child manipulated a bracelet (B) made of eight wooden beads consisting of five big beads (A) and three small beads (A'). The bracelet was hidden behind a screen. The first questions related to the form, material, number and size of the beads. The experimenter then asked about the inclusion (A<B): "Are all the small beads made of wood? Are all the big beads made of wood? If you make a bracelet with all the wooden beads (B) and another with all the big beads (A) which will be the larger? Are there more wooden beads or more big beads in the bracelet?", etc. Children were classified according to the criteria established by Piaget and Szeminska (1941) to justify class-inclusion as a concrete operation. Again, the RH group (4 to 12 years old, N = 62) performed better with the left hand (p = 0.0027) but in the LH group this difference was not significant (4 to 8 years old, N = 92).

Probabilities
Thinking about probabilities implies a formal balance between favorable cases vs possible cases. A tactile test for the quantification of probabilities was adapted from Piaget and Inhelder (1956). Using only one hand in a blind situation as before, a set of smooth wooden cubes S was compared with a set of rough cubes R. For instance: one S and four R were compared with two S and four R. In which set is there a higher probability of picking up a rough cube R at the first attempt? A correct answer implies the comparison of pairs in the example above $(4/5) > (4/6)$ where the higher probability of picking up an R is in the first set. A large number of different probabilities was presented to 224 RH adolescents (12 to 18 years old). No LH subjects were submitted to this test. In the RH group we detected a higher performance in formal operations in those using the left hand (p=0.045). As in the other logical tasks (conservation of substance and class-inclusion), the right hemisphere seems to play a key role as a relay of the information which will be fully processed by the left hemisphere. I am now entitled to ask what happens in the case of the right hemisphere being removed?

In the first place, it could be shown that for "concrete operations" such as class-inclusion or conservation of substance, and for "formal operations" such as probabilities, the right-handed children who used their left hands, thus activating their right hemispheres, performed at a significantly higher level than the group using their right hands and left hemispheres! The inverse phenomenon occurred in concrete spatial operations such as the conservation of length of a rod; the group who used their right hands, thus activating

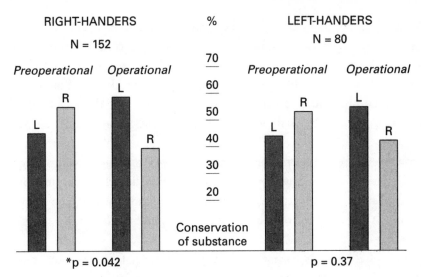

RIGHT-HANDERS N = 152

LEFT-HANDERS N = 80

%

Preoperational Operational

Preoperational Operational

*p = 0.042

p = 0.37

Conservation of substance

Figure 6.1   Distribution of pre-operational and operational performances on the Piagetian task of conservation of substance with different hands L: left, R: right, in right-handers and left-handers.

their left hemispheres, attained a more advanced level of spatial reasoning. However, no significant difference in cognitive performance was found in the left-handed group, irrespective of which hand and therefore, which brain hemisphere was used. The reason for this may be that they have a larger bilateral cortical representation (Satz, 1979). What is the explanation for this intriguing result? We know that the information gathered by the left hand goes first to the right hemisphere and then reaches the left hemisphere in a second step via the corpus callosum, and vice versa. The amazing conclusion was that different neuronal paths favor different (logical or spatial) kinds of operational thinking and were perfectly crossed in the right-handed group. For instance,

(a) in the logical tests of conservation of substance, class inclusion and probabilities, the subjects attained concrete thinking at higher operative levels with the sequence: left hand > right hemisphere > left hemisphere.

(b) in the spatial test of conservation of length, by contrast, the subjects attained the best cognitive performance with the sequence: right hand > left hemisphere > right hemisphere.

We posited the hypothesis that the dominant left hemisphere (associated mainly with logical processing) made use of the preceding contribution of the minor right hemisphere (associated more with spatial processing) for the logical tasks. Conversely, the right hemisphere would make use of the left one for spatial processing. If I interpret Minsky's theory of the society of the mind correctly, the crossed route would activate a larger number of "agents," a good strategy for the developing mind. But when a stable cognitive stage (concrete or formal operations) is reached, a few "managers" will suffice to do the entire job. If the right brain is a childish brain then the left brain should manage the higher Piagetian levels in the tasks we are discussing on its own, without the help of the right brain. We now have the opportunity to test this hypothesis.

As we have seen, Nico reached the Piagetian stage of conservation of substance when he was six years old. What happens if we repeat the test two years later, but this time in a blind situation? The change from vision to touch is crucial here: instead of seeing the transformation of the ball into a sausage with his own eyes, he will be forced to rely solely on the tactile and proprioceptive feedback from his hands. The right hand is not disabled and connects normally to the left hemisphere. Following the right hemispherectomy, however, no crossed paths exist from the left hand, only some relatively minor ipsilateral connections to the left brain remain (Benecke *et al.*, 1991, Adelson *et al.*, 1995). As previously mentioned, Nico still has some restricted movement in his left hand but his stereognosia is impaired. When asked to identify some familiar solid objects (a key, a spoon, a fork) behind a screen with his left hand, he had great difficulty and gave no correct answers. However, with his right hand he immediately identified the objects correctly. What is your conjecture about the result of this tactile version of the Piagetian test? Let us try to apply our compensatory analysis. First, if the left hemisphere fully compensates for the loss of the right one, then no deviation from the cognitive norm will be observed. The half-brained child who acquired the concept of conservation of substance two years earlier would thus have no difficulty in replicating the same reasoning in the new blind setting as when the tactile information passed from the right hand to the left hemisphere. The main contralateral connections to the left hemisphere would suffice to give reliable information on the transformation of the ball of clay. But would the minor ipsilateral

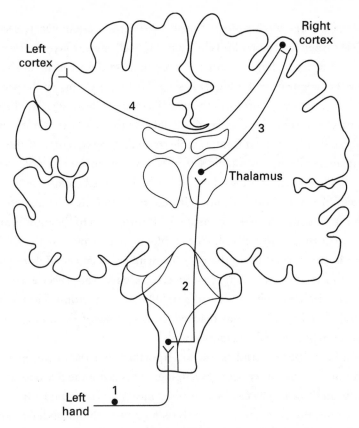

Figure 6.2   Crossed pathways. 1 Dorsal funiculus, 2 Crossing lemniscal fibers, ventral thalamic nucleus. 3 Somesthesic projection system. 4 Inter-hemispheric fibers, callosum.

pathways from the left hand to the left hemisphere convey the same kind of information? The prediction from compensatory analysis would say no. In effect, Nico gave a perfect response to the Piagetian task of conservation of substance using his right hand, but not with his left hand! This is exactly the inverse situation to the group of normal children who showed a higher cognitive performance with their left hands. In other words, cortical compensation is fully developed for concrete tasks which reach the left brain via a crossed main path but not via the ipsilateral connection.

For the moment this example suffices for our purpose. In fact, the standard visual situation is not equivalent to the blind tests for many reasons. In the first place, it is known that most of the Piagetian tasks are subject to a systematic delay when tested on blind children (Hatwell *et al.*, 1985). In the second place, vision has a larger cortical representation than touch. In the third place, every cognitive test is highly susceptible to any change in the presentation of the task, i.e. a shift from the visual to the tactile mode is not insignificant and may produce a "décalage" – a delay in the acquisition of the notion being tested. Therefore, it is impossible to predict the outcome of the cognitive processing in the new tactile setting, even with normal (double brained) children. How much more so then with a half-brained child with hemianopia, hemiplegia and only a minor ipsilateral connection to his left hemisphere? In this case there is no transfer of information to the right brain and all the processing (whether visual or tactile) must take place in the left hemisphere. In the normal brain the right hemisphere is activated in the logical process of the conservation of substance, but seems to have been entirely substituted by the left one in the case of a right hemispherectomy. The fact is that with only one brain Nico has reached the last stage of the conservation of substance in both visual and tactile modes.

Brain lateralization studies are so important that they take up a whole chapter of contemporary neuropsychology. This is not the place to summarize these findings as they can be consulted in several recent and authoritative publications. But compensatory analysis might enrich our understanding of the subject,[3] particularly when we consider the opposing views of cognitive modularity and constructivism, the paradigms of Noam Chomsky and Jean Piaget as expressed in the celebrated 1975 Royaumont debate between the two scientists (Piatelli-Palmarini, 1979, 1994). Chomsky emphasizes the need to study cognitive structures (particularly language) as "mental organs" in the same way that we study any physical organ such as the heart or the brain itself. He explicitly refutes the Piagetian constructivist approach of a sequence of cognitive stages developing in complexity from the sensory-motor schemes to the higher formal operations. He thinks, for instance, that the mental organ of language has an ontogenetic as well as philogenetic history which follows the genetic program of the species. Piaget on the other hand, affirms that "only the functioning of intelligence has a hereditary basis but the production of (cognitive) structures is given by the organization of successive actions upon the objects".

Now we can add some new results that were unavailable at the time of that debate. They stress the importance of the epigenetic component in the brain and of cognitive development. As we have reported, the existence of only half a brain does not prevent the development of Piagetian mental operations in the expected order. As distinct from the case of many organic deficits, where only a portion of the specific biological tissue develops fully, there is no such thing as an "incomplete mental organ." Nor can we find any evidence of faulty logical reasoning when the hemispherectomized subject is duly submitted to cognitive testing. Instead we observe fully fledged reasoning, never half reasoning with half a brain! It is well known that during embriogenesis and immediately following birth a significant destruction of neurons occurs, a physiological process which has been described by Jean-Pierre Changeux (1983) as "une hécatombe neuronale" – a neuronal devastation. What then should be the term which expresses the elimination of thousands of millions of neurons and synapses by hemispherectomy! It is hard to imagine any Chomskian "mental organ" surviving such surgery. How could the functions of the right brain be assimilated into the left hemisphere without a radical reorganization of the neural networks? The idea of a kind of "modular cloning" within the brain seems no less unreasonable than that of right and left copies of the same modular unit or mental organ which can be activated when required. In my view the central Piagetian (1967, 1975) idea of cognitive equilibrium offers a better explanation for the radical reorganization of mental processes following a functional hemispherectomy. This is the idea of an equilibrium between assimilation and accommodation, between the subsystems of a system within a new global system ("équilibration majorante"). In Nico we have an extreme case of cognitive re-equilibration following a massive neuronal perturbation. Moreover, there is some recent physiological evidence to suggest that Piagetian cognitive cycles of accommodation and assimilation can be related to cyclic cortical activity (Thatcher, 1998, Fischer, 1997).

New dynamic models of cognitive and cortical growth can now be tested following the removal of a hemisphere. We would certainly need to know if, as in the case of hemispherectomized animals, the remaining hemisphere uses a greater number of neurons in order to compensate for the lost hemisphere (Adelson et al.,1995). But metabolic constraints will certainly limit the number of neurons that can be simultaneously active. We can conclude that the successful activation of alternative neurocognitive networks as a result of hemispherectomy reflects the amazing plasticity and redundancy of cerebral connectivity. It reflects the enormous power of the human brain wide web. Our double brain is undoubtedly the inner frontier of knowledge.

7   Brain, education, and development

Fabricando fabricemur

DIDACTICA MAGNA, 1640
JAN AMOS COMENIUS

This chapter has a distant source in one of the founding fathers of modern pedagogy, the Czech theologian Jan Amos Comenius (1592–1670). His proposition was "to learn to write in writing, to sing in singing, to think in thinking." He also introduced an interesting correspondence between mind, brain, and thinking (mens, cerebrum, ratio) on the one hand, and hands, activity, and artistic skill (manus, operatio, artes) on the other. Three centuries later Jean Piaget (1957) reinterpreted this outdated concept in the modern "act and construct" framework of developmental psychology and progressive education: "understanding of the rule derives from the retroactive organization of examples already utilized in spontaneous practice." Today the way forward for the education of future generations is two-fold – the digital web which connects people and institutions across the planet, and the brain web of new synaptic connections made inside our heads in the process of learning. We are talking here about an extremely large scale of interactions, both internal and external, a very complex system which is still difficult to imagine, compute or manage for current educational purposes. Consequently, this final chapter should be interpreted as a preliminary sketch of that delicate process of amazing complexity I call neuroeducation.[1]

I will try to describe briefly how brain, education and development are

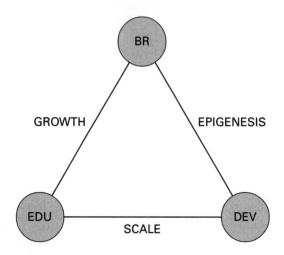

Figure 7.1   BRED. Brain, education, and development

linked in a triad I call BRED. A half-brained child gave me the unique opportunity to reflect on this topic and to monitor some precise pedagogical inter-
ventions in this new field. But BRED should also be treated as an area of
knowledge in itself and as a wider program of action that can hopefully lead
to the enrichment of many lives in our global society.

Figure 7.1 may help to understand the new concept of BRED: BRain, Education and Development. The nodes BR, EDU, DEV are represented as the
points of a triangle and the sides represent the links: BR-EDU, EDU-DEV,
DEV-BR. To each link I propose to "paste" the observed neurocognitive phenomena and the main concepts involved. For the sake of brevity I have chosen
six links (from a larger collection) which I have studied extensively in other
contexts, and which were selected to fit our study of a half-brained mind.

I firmly believe that the education of an hemispherectomized child can
open new perspectives on the way we understand human nature and the
nature of education itself.

Transitions and the link between education and the brain
Education is a widely inclusive cultural phenomenon which accepts all cate-
gories of individuals and seeks to overcome all kinds of obstacles, especially
those which relate to physical and mental disabilities. Those teachers who are
dedicated to so-called "special education" know well how much pedagogical

Table 7.1 *BRED links*

BRED	*phenomena*	*concepts*
EDU-BR	learning curves	transitions
EDU-DEV	micro/macro	change of scale
DEV-BR	compensation	epigenetic growth

effort is dedicated to the training of precise, controlled skills. Over a period of more than fifteen years I have worked thousands of hours endeavouring to help such children (and their families) to deal with their disabilities. Nico the first hemispherectomized child I met in my whole career, was a new challenge for everybody. To help him we put together an interdisciplinary team of teachers, psychologists, and technicians. We met regularly at school in a monthly seminar to assess Nico's schooling in every possible field of activity. In addition I had regular conversations with Nico's parents and, of course, many opportunities to work with him either in a group situation, or individually, both at school and at home. From the outset we have kept a detailed record of his school work and have videotaped some of his activities. These records allow me to affirm today that his early epileptic trouble and his right hemispherectomy have not – so far – given rise to any specific impediment to Nico's learning process. On the contrary, he learns at the same pace as his schoolmates and he follows a normal developmental trend. But of course Nico's education needs careful and responsible supervision in order to detect any sign of trouble as soon as possible. We cannot take for granted that he will continue to learn and develop without major problems. He attends a large, busy school with hundreds of pupils and a great diversity of requirements and we are ready to implement new educational strategies if at any stage he should begin to show signs of stress under the ever increasing institutional strain, or fall behind his classmates. All the signs, however, indicate that Nico is performing up to his own and our expectations.

We can now explore the first cell of Table 7.1, the learning process, and for this purpose we can take the example of Nico's written language. As I have stated, his written output does not differ from the norm for his age. It might

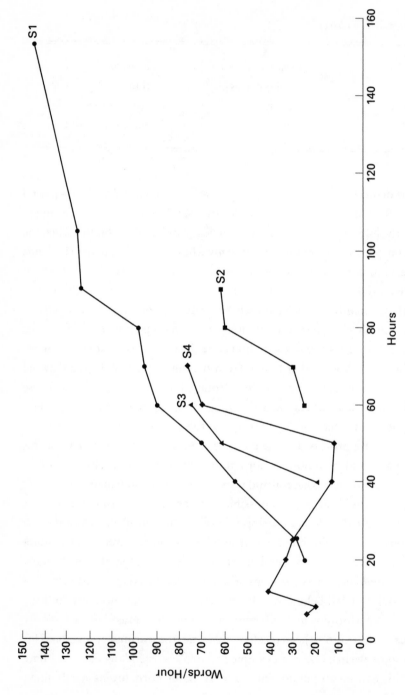

Figure 7.2 Learning curves for writing skills. S1. Age 18: mild mental retardation, S2. Age 20: borderline, spina bifida, quadriplegia, S3. Age 17: Down's syndrome (trisomy 21) and S4. Age 16: autism with visceral and somatic malformations.

be useful however, to compare his computer writing skills with those of some other brain disabled subjects. For them the writing process develops very slowly, a feature that will allow us to make a more precise analysis of the respective learning curves with a word processor in general. Figure 7.2 shows the learning curves with a word processor of four handicapped youths. After a latent period which varies from two to forty hours of weekly training, the disabled student is capable of at most twenty written words in a one hour session (mostly as a copy of some printed text). We can take this as a turning point. Then a most remarkable "explosion" in the quality (decrease in the number of errors) and quantity of writing (increase in the number of words per hour) takes place until a plateau is reached. All the subjects show a comparable acceleration in their written output (similar slopes in the learning curves) after a specific time-delay. To sum up, these sigmoidal learning curves are composed of three segments: first, a latency period which may extend to dozens of hours of practice, second, a clear transition with a very steep segment of improved performance, third, a plateau is reached showing a stabilized skill. This kind of non-linear development of a simple skill is very common, as has been described in detail (Fischer and Rose, 1994, 1998; Thatcher et al.,1997). What is important here is the rapidity of the change in the transitional phase, where we observe a similar slope in all four cases. This abrupt increase in output is accompanied by a simultaneous dramatic decrease in the number of errors (misspelt words), which in some cases drops to under 10 per cent after initially representing over 80 per cent of the total written production! This abrupt increase in efficiency seems to be a general neurocognitive phenomenon during the acquisition of many skills. My conjecture is that this leap forward can be linked to the opening of new neural pathways in the brain.

A simple explanation for the exceptionally long time it takes for these handicapped persons to acquire new abilities is that their brains need a longer period of activation to trigger a new way of doing things. The clinical difficulty is to keep the subject active during the protracted and tedious latency period, the duration of which can inhibit further learning, either because of lack of motivation and positive feedback, or even because the subject's consistently poor results cause the demotivation of the instructor. It can often seem as if the training never reaches the threshold capable of "opening" new cognitive paths in the brain and building new neural net-works. We can say that the first changes take place after approximately ten hours of practice and that a plateau can be attained at around 100 hours. But a new scaling factor can be triggered and a new explosion in written output observed after about 1,000 hours of computer work. This final spurt enables some disabled students to look for jobs as clerks, but few subjects stay long enough to reach this second threshold. We may interpret the accelerated segment of written performance – and the correlated decrease in errors – as a behavioral sign of the "opening" in the brain of new cognitive paths for writing. Logarithmic scales are known to represent psychophysical phenom-ena. At this point they help us to establish a functional link between the brain and learning. The concept that sheds the most light on the whole learning sit-uation is that of "transition" – the abrupt change in the underlying dynamic of the learning process from one stable stage (few words, many errors) to another stable stage (many words, few errors). There is a whole branch of mathematics known as catastrophe theory, developed by René Thom (1972) which might be applied to model this kind of bi-stable behavior. The abrupt transition from one level of written performance to the other can be inter-preted as a "cusp" in the mathematical sense of the theory of catastrophes, but we need more experiments to test the model in greater detail. The catas-trophe theory became fashionable at the end of the 1970s when I became engaged in that topic too (Battro,1976; Rozestraten, Battro and Santos Andrade, 1976). Now, with the new angle on dynamics and bifurcations of neural networks it is surfacing again with some interesting results in experi-mental psychology (Wang and Blum,1995).

We never subjected Nico to an exhausting one hour session on a word pro-cessor. But from his day-to-day records at school (over a period of three years) we observed a steady increase in the quantity and quality of his writing; a very low number of errors (less than 10 per cent) from the outset (copy) and a format of short messages of about forty words (free production, letters, com-ments, etc.). This would represent an estimated output of more than 300 words per hour, double that of the best 18-year-old pupil from our former study. We can infer from these data that Nico's latency period was very brief and that the transition to a plateau was abrupt. He has now attained a satis-factory written output but his typing is comparatively slower than the actual (hand-written) production of many of his classmates. This quantitative difference could become greater in the future and might have some detrimental educational consequences. However, things may improve now because of Nico's growing use of email, which in itself merits comment.

For a child, the fact of communicating via the Internet signifies a qualitative cognitive change (as it is for every one of us). I am convinced that the rehabilitation process of a handicapped person can be enriched by regular email contact. I must say that this is a new kind of professional (medical or psychological) tool, which for some reason is underestimated by my colleagues. For instance, most computers in hospital are operated by healthy adults. Very few patients have access to them, fewer still if those patients are children. However, when this technology becomes accessible, it can change the quality of life of the disabled user. I began to explore the beneficial effects of email with deaf children when computers were first introduced in schools in the early 1980s and I extended the idea of networking to many other disabled students as well. Via the network we were able to communicate easily with a deaf adolescent who designed all the computer graphics for our book about "discommunications," an essay on the use of computers with the deaf (Battro and Denham, 1987). Its social impact aside, email offered all of them the unique opportunity to combine the syntactic, semantic and pragmatic dimensions of language in one single act of communication through the Web. And this is essential for education. I always try to maintain a regular email exchange with my former students with disabilities and I certainly recommend this professional practice. Some of them are still sending emails after more than ten years. It is a very gratifying experience indeed for the teacher and the student!

Formal education has traditionally been confined to the communication which takes place within the school walls. Today circumstances have changed and students and teachers can enjoy and benefit from a wider horizon of communication through the Web. We have also empowered Nico's communication capabilities by means of a sustained digital link. With these resources we have opened up a new world to him and his whole class. Initial results have been very exciting, although it is too early to predict the scope of this email activity in the long term. But in a year's time I fully expect the whole class to have established a regular digital habit, as is frequently the case when the school provides "email for all" at an early age. The next step will be to develop the necessary skills to surf the Web. I must confess my great joy when I receive a message from Nico, an event which I await daily with a mixture of admiration and expectation. We have established some ground rules for send/reply operations and we respect a commitment to keep up regular exchanges. We have so many things to share! At this point in time it is hard to imagine the life of a half-brained child as a young man, but I believe this digital habit will grow as he does.

The change of scale and the link between education and development

This is a more general topic and I shall follow a different route – from concepts to facts. Education can be described as an intervention in the course of mental development. Both are closely linked and modern theory and practice provide a vast amount of evidence for their strong correlation over a person's entire life span. Jean Piaget was one of the most prominent advocates of establishing a progressive education based on the different stages of human development. He recognized Comenius as the founding father of the idea, but progressive education seems to be as beset with difficulties today as it was in the seventeenth century. Some optimists, and I belong to this category, believe that we are on the verge of a sea change in the old educational paradigm because of the massive impact of computers and communications on society. In fact we are about to see a radical change in the "scale" of education. And this lies at the core of our discussion.

I know that the question of scale, of the change of magnitude in a system, is extremely complex. In education we must face this question from the outset. As a matter of fact education is very sensitive to quantitative changes, and every teacher, administrator or minister of education knows this. In the first place, a mere increase in the amount of equipment or human resources does not ensure a qualitative leap forward in learning. In the second place, education seems to be "scale dependent." This explains why it is impossible to apply a possible success in a restricted learning environment to a broader one. In other words pedagogical intervention is valid only in the specific scale in which it has been tested. Unlike engineers who can simulate the behavior of a river in a scale model of a dam, educators cannot predict the outcome of a national program from a well monitored model in a few experimental schools. Education is not scalable in the sense that hydrodynamics is. In this context we have performed a wide variety of experiments with children concerning some Piagetian cognitive invariants using different scales. We discovered, for instance, that the psychogenetic construction of the 1–1 correspondence and of the projective lines were scale-dependent, the conservation of surfaces and the axiom of distance, on the contrary, were scale-independent (Battro *et al.*, 1976, 1977). For example, the acquisition of the concept of 1–1 correspondence between large objects (such as real cars and real trees) is delayed in time compared with the ordinary tests using small objects (eggs and egg-cups). A systematic study of this kind of significant cognitive scale-shifts should be reconsidered in the era of globalization. Scale too, therefore, should be a matter of pedagogical concern.

Micro education and macro education seem to be altogether different disciplines. Each node in the BRED system has specific internal scales. There is a micro-EDU in the short learning process of a simple skill (eg. click and drag a computer mouse) and a macro-EDU in the long learning process of a domain (eg. musical composition). There is a micro-DEV in problem solving (eg. recursion in the Tower of Hanoi task) and a macro-DEV in geometric concepts (eg. from simple topological to elaborate Euclidean thinking). Each of these levels corresponds to a specific space and time scale and they can be mixed in a very complex manner. A similar imbrication of levels has been reported in Chapter 2 in relation to the BR node (microcycles of brain growth within macrocycles or tiers of cortical reorganization). The change of scale may modify the way we teach a half-brained child. Nico is being educated in a private school equipped with a wealth of computers and digital networks, a television production studio, online videoconferencing facilities, and the like. He is totally immersed in a digital environment. We have observed that this rich informational milieu is providing a crucial prosthetic support, especially for his writing skills. In years to come he will be using many other digital school facilities to develop a larger array of skills. We have already described the nature of a "digital education" (Battro and Denham, 1997) and it will suffice for our purpose to reflect briefly on the impact of these technologies on the education of a half-brained child. We are dealing here with the new frontiers of knowledge in the digital world of the future.

First, we know that one of the principal properties of digital systems is their astonishing "scalability," we can add more and more computers and optic fibers to a network without altering its nature. The digital world has no frontiers and is expanding smoothly in a seamless network that will soon cover the whole planet. At school the profound changes from a simple local network to the World Wide Web, from intranet to Internet, from a BBS to a home page, are akin to the growth of a living system. Let me recount my experience at a school where everybody made very intensive use of the local digital network. One day the number of students and teachers using the Internet reached 1,000. They were exchanging the same kind of messages as before but on a global scale! This abrupt and impressive change of scale of many degrees of magnitude was clear to all of them. The same digital behavior pattern is being repeated in an increasing number of schools around the world. Nico is extremely fortunate to have been born at the end of the twentieth century, when a well trained half-brained person will certainly receive his fair share of the formidable expansion of knowledge which the growing digital world has to offer.

Second, I would like to emphasize some of the invariant properties of many of the functional changes which link a change of scale in education with individual mental development. For a half-brained child such as Nico, as for any "double-brained" child, it is important to feel at home when facing tasks of increasing difficulty, even when some of these imply a change of scale. A pedagogically well designed task will convey some functional anchors as well as some structural analogies which may be recognized as invariants, despite the increasing complexity of the whole problem. Let me give an example from a different domain, that of urban design. For many years I have been working on the cognition and perception of urban space by children and adults and I had the good fortune to work with the late Kevin Lynch (1960,1979), a pioneer in the field. With a large team of psychologists and architects in several towns we established the developmental trends in the psychological representation of the urban features that make up the general pattern of a place: borders (i.e. a river), zones (a park), paths (a street), landmarks (a church), nodes (a road crossing). The children were asked to go round a large part of their own town and then build a maquette, a scale model of the place, and also to make some drawings. We discovered that the representation of the urban plan was made in stages; the paths were established first, the landmarks last. And most interestingly, when we asked them to visit and reproduce a small public park instead of a large urban space, we discovered that the same pattern from paths to landmarks was repeated. In this particular instance, a part of the town, a public place, was itself composed of borders, zones, paths, landmarks, and nodes, just as in the town as a whole! These five features act as invariants or cognitive anchors in the change of scale (Battro and Ellis, 1989). We interpreted this cognitive phenomenon as an example of "self-similarity," a central concept of Benoit Mandelbrot's (1997) mathematical theory of fractals. These mathematical objects can be self-similar, i.e. a part of an object conserves some of the properties of the whole object. For instance, when we inspect a coast in detail we can observe bays and capes, but if we proceed further, with a finer measurement, we find other similar (but smaller) bays and capes in a shorter section of the same coast. We can continue at smaller and smaller scales and the complexity will continue to grow (bays inside bays inside bays . . .). This is a restricted geographical example of recursion but if properly extended to a mathematical curve the complexity and length of the coast line will grow endlessly. There are many interesting models of this sort of recursive self-similar curves (Koch curves, for example). I believe that fractals may help to analyze some theoretical questions in our BRED model too. In particular those questions related to the micro and macro levels. For instance, how do we manage to go from an individual micro-development to a collective macro-education? or from macro-development to a micro-learning process? We must recognize that we are still in trouble when dealing with changes of scale and self-similarity problems in education and psychology, but there are some new developments in the most advanced neurosciences, as is the case with fractal strategies for neural networking scaling (Lister, 1995).

This notion of spatial invariance can be taken as a metaphor for many kinds of cognitive changes of scale during learning. The same invariants frequently crop up at both the macro and micro levels. For instance, when children transfer their writing skills from simple word processing for homework to higher levels of communication, such as sending messages on the Internet, an important cognitive change of scale takes place but the basic digital skill (writing sentences on a computer) remains invariant. The scale shift, however, is considerable. The first task is at the level of a micro-development, the second can open the door to long-distance education, a macro-educational level. Shifting from one level to the other, changing cognitive scales, is an essential activity in education. Nico is now engaged in this ever empowering practice through email, thanks to the fortunate choice of a school in which digital education is bringing about the spread of new global links to develop the potential of each student.

Epigenetic growth and the links between the brain and mental development
Epigenesis is the opposite of preformation. It can be studied in the development of an organism interacting with the environment. There is a developmental path to be followed, a "chreod" in Conrad H. Waddington's (1974) terminology. But this dynamic process can suffer all kinds of disturbances, both natural and artificial. Experimental embryology is based on the ability to provoke and monitor these disturbances. Waddington proposed a dynamic theory according to which some disturbances in the system can be corrected by a procedure known as homeo-rhesis. This is defined as a regulated flow through the basins of an "epigenetic landscape," with hills and valleys, the unstable repulsors and stable attractors of the dynamic system. These dynamic notions are also very useful in the study of neural development, where hereditary and acquired factors are closely interwoven. Jean-Pierre Changeux has defined the notion of a "genetic envelope" as the frontier between the invariant characteristics submitted to the strict determinism of genes and the characteristics submitted to phenotypic variability (in Piatelli-Palmarini, 1979). There is a huge amount of evidence relating to epigenetic phenomena in the nervous system. For example, at the molecular level the synapses are constantly renewed in the neuromuscular juncture of the embryo (every twenty hours) and also in the adult (every eleven days). The whole brain is submitted to an important epigenetic regulation by nervous activity (Arbib *et al.*, 1998).

The BR-DEV link is essentially an epigenetic link. Jean Piaget was perhaps the first psychologist to have made the transfer of the epigenetic model from biological evolution to cognitive development in a systematic way. His example has been followed by others, and it can be said that the study of epigenetic mechanisms is at the cutting edge of one of the most advanced areas of neurocognition. Hemispherectomy studies may also profit from these advances. The surgical removal of the right cortex in particular, as in Nico's case, represents a key test for the epigenetic reorganization of the left cortex. And this in turn implies a revision of our theories about the neural processes involved in the acquisition and growth of human knowledge. Piaget called genetic epistemology the study "of the mechanisms of the growth of knowledge" and he made a distinction between restricted and generalized genetic epistemology. The former includes "all psychogenetic research or historico-critical research about the methods of the growth of knowledge, to the extent that it is based on a system of reference constituted by the state of knowledge existing at the moment of observation." In the latter "the reference system is itself included in the genetic or in the historical process which has to be studied" (Piaget, 1950). In this sense, perhaps the study of the epigenetic mechanisms of the developing brain will lead to a new "epigenetic epistemology."

I am convinced that any progress in the theory of knowledge will profit in a fundamental manner from the epigenetic study of brain development. We saw a reconstruction of the hemispherectomy performed on Nico some five years ago on a virtual reality workbench. Using similar technology we can imagine a digital brain atlas which will be able to simulate the continuous growth of the different structures of the nervous system – fibers, nuclei, gyri, cortices. This description will illustrate the neural developmental curve from birth (or before) to full brain growth (and its subsequent regression), in short, the complete arc of life, particularly the segment which spans the school years when a significant proportion of the brain's growth takes place. I must say that in the course of my research I became increasingly aware of the amazing changes in the shape and size of a child's head which we usually take for granted because of the overall growth of the body. Pediatricians and anthropologists have studied this fact for decades but few educators have assimilated the profound consequences of this phenomenon from the point of view of the growing neural web inside the skull during schooling. Should we wait for a twenty-first century D'Arcy Wentworth Thompson (1952) striving to describe the "growth and form" of neural structures? Neuro-education certainly needs a good map of the schooled brain in different scales of anatomical detail. It is worth noting that as yet the field of current brain imaging has provided little information on the developing brain. And we can even imagine a corresponding dynamic atlas of the growing brain in which the location of the most important cognitive processes will be shown as they evolve. We certainly need to map this new "epigenetic landscape" but this is no easy task and should be included in a far reaching BRED program.

My thesis that "the half-brain is a new brain" will also need rigorous epigenetic study, at all possible levels, from the micro-architecture of synaptogenesis to the macro-connectivity of emergent neural networks. I am aware that in this book I have only drawn a rough sketch of the epigenetic neurocognitive landscape of a half-brained person, but I hope many others will go more deeply into what I have explored superficially. With the help of team work we should begin to unravel the marvels of the amazing reconstruction of the brain which I have been so fortunate to study.

Notes

1 **The heart is in the brain**

1 The book *Education and the brain,* edited by Jeanne S. Chall and Allan F. Mirsky
(1978), is one of the rare publications in recent times that deals explicitly with the
subject I now call "neuroeducation." At that time *The National Society for the
Study of Education NSSE,* founded a commission on *Education and the Brain*
with such distinguished scholars in both fields as Jeanne S. Chall, Allan F. Mirsky,
Richard Held, Jerome Kagan, Horace W. Magoun, Richard L. Thompson,
Sheldon H. White and Merlin C. Wittrock. We can also find some remarkable
insights in the same vein in the last century. A professor of neurology of the University of Chicago, Henry Herbert Donaldson, wrote a very interesting book *The
growth of the brain: A study of the nervous system in relation to education*
(1896). He began his study, a century ago, with the following words "we are told
that this age is one of nervous strain . . ."

I think it would be fruitful today to continue the work these pioneers have
started. The new master concentration directed by Kurt W. Fischer at Harvard
Graduate School of Education: *Mind, Brain and Education, MBE* is an answer to
that challenge.

2 The study of the damaged brain has been for many scientists a platform for
philosophical reflexion. The eminent German neurologist, Kurt Goldstein
(1878–1965), delivered the 1938–39 William James Lecture at Harvard with the
title *Human nature in the light of psychopathology* (1940). It must be said that
Goldstein's classical text *Der Aufbau des Organismus* (1934) was very influential
on European phenomenology, in particular on the work of Maurice Merleau
Ponty. I had the chance to audit his teaching at the Collège de France when I was at

the Laboratoire de Psychologie Expérimentale et Comparée at Sorbonne with Paul Fraisse (1958–60). I can also say that I considered myself a remote follower of Goldstein during my medical education at the University of Buenos Aires (1952–57). I must now confess that I reread his book forty years later during the writing of this book, searching for philosophical inspiration, but the ideas that excited me as a young physician have aged badly. A caveat for the author – and to those who may dare to read this book in the year 2040!

But, *feci quod potui, faciant meliora potentes . . .*

3   The bibliography on hemispherectomized patients is very large. The first medical reports came from L'Hermite (1928) and Dandy (1928). Other interesting historical antecedents are Gardner (1933) and McKenzie (1938).

For recent medical follow-up studies see Byrne and Gates(1987), Green et al, (1988), Davies *et al.* (1993), Lindsay *et al.* (1987), Peacock *et al.* (1996). For cognitive disturbances in child epilepsy see Deonna (1998).

From the point of view of neuropsychology see Bach y Rita (1980), Damasio, Lima and Damasio (1975), Day and Ulatowska (1979). In an older review Gott (1973) describes the results of a large battery of cognitive tests after surgery. See also McFie (1961). A very useful general summary is Vargha-Khadem and Polkey (1992).

For visual functions see Kohn and Dennis (1974), King *et al.* (1996).

For auditive functions see Poirier *et al.* (1994).

For language see Basser (1962) who reports 113 cases.

Kohn and Dennis (1974), Dennis and Kohn (1975), Dennis and Whitaker (1976, 1977), Whitaker and Ojeman (1977), Dennis (1980), Dennis *et al.* (1981), Odgen (1988), Patterson *et al.* (1989), Stark *et al.*(1995, 1997), Vargha-Khadem *et al.* (1991), Zaidel,(1973, 1980, 1981).

From the point of view of the recovery of sensorimotor functions after hemispherectomy, see Benecke *et al.* (1991) and Müller *et al.* (1991). They report that "an astonishing motor repertoire is preserved by remaining projections." The major candidate for this reorganization is the premotor reticulo-spinal pathway. The authors give a useful list of sixty-four references on hemispherectomy and hemidecortication.

4   Interesting references of brain models on the Internet are:
the University of Southern California Brain Project
www-hbp.usc.edu/HBP/models/
and the Brain Map produced by the University of Texas
http://ric.uthscsa.edu/services

Also some major publications can be reached at the Web, like the *Journal of Contemporary Neurology:* www.mitpress.mit.edu/neurology.html

The progressive interdisciplinary approach for complex phenomena is revealed by the increasing number of co-authors in a scientific paper. The largest number I have counted in a single publication on cognitive neurosciences is twelve co-authors, (Silbersweig et al, 1995) still one order of magnitude less than some of the most recent papers on experimental physics, for example. It can be expected that our discipline will continue to grow fast and will require a larger integration of experts in different fields, in particular with the introduction of new and more powerful non-invasive brain imaging technologies. In the same line of thought it is interesting to see that two major recent textbooks edited by Arbib (1995) and Gazzaniga (1995) are well above the 1,000 printed pages and include dozens of collaborations! In the future even a single-case analysis in cognitive neurosciences, such as this book, would require a very large group of experts. A change of scale quite difficult to imagine by our current standards indeed, but I don't think contemporary "romantic science," in Luria's sense, should be incompatible with a strong collaborative interplay among many experts.

2   Sculpting a new brain

1   We certainly need the help of the most advanced neuroanatomy to know the actual order of magnitude of the number of functional units of the brain, neurons, and synapses. The experts give quite different figures. My idea of talking in terms of Meganeuron, Giganeuron, Teraneuron or Petasynapse may seem presumptuous, but I think it will become useful, when someday the technical notion of brainpower becomes operational. For more details see Blinkov and Glezer(1968). Schütz (1995) estimates between 7×10^{10} and 8×10^{10} neurons in the whole human brain, 5×10^{10} in the cortex, 10^6 (1 Meganeuron in my terms) in the thalamus, 10^8 fibers in corpus callosum and 10^{14} synapses. Edelman and Mountcastle (1978) report 5×10^9 neurons in the neocortex (5 Giganeuron), Churchland (1996) shares the common view of the brain having 10^{11} neurons and 10^{14} synapses. These figures are one order of magnitude less than the Teraneuron and Petasynapse I have given. But other authors confirm the value of 10^{15} synapses, see Changeux and Ricoeur (1998). See also Evrad and Minkowski (1989), Gilles *et al.* (1983). Huttenlocher (1984, 1990), Lenneberg (1967), Rosenzweig (1979).

2   Fischer's views on cognitive skills and brain development are reported in Fischer, K. W. and Rose, S. P. (1994, 1996), Fischer and Bidell (1998). He defines skill as a "capacity to act in an organized way in a specific context" (p. 478). Skills are

context specific, self-organizing and organized in multilevel hierarchies. Skills follow a regular sequence of changes during mental development: 1) single sets of skills, 2) mappings between sets, 3) systems between mappings, and 4) systems of systems. He hypothesized that "one cycle of these changes involves movement through one developmental level or stage"(1996, p. 272). At each level, "connectivity in the right hemisphere contracts during the cycle . . . and connectivity in the left hemisphere expands" (1996, p. 272–3). This hypothesis is compelling because "it provides an appropriate mechanism for the growth of neural networks at each developmental level" (*ibid.*)

3 Compensatory analysis

1   The main European sources of lesion analysis in contemporary philosophy were Goldstein (1934) and Merleau-Ponty (1942, 1944). See also Popper and Eccles (1977) for a continuation of the classical debate, where hemispherectomy is (briefly) discussed. A fresh view on lesion analysis can be found in the recent dialogue between the French philosopher Paul Ricoeur and the neuroscientist Jean-Pierre Changeux (1998). The American counterpart is now blooming, Bickle (1998), Clark (1996), Churchland (1986), Churchland (1996), Graham and Lynn Stephens (1997), Crick (1994), Solso (1997), Edelman (1992), Koch and Davis (1994).

2   The main reference is Geshwind and Galaburda (1987). A remarkable analysis of these findings is given in Winner (1996). See her chapter 6: The biology of giftedness. For a critical evaluation of the GGS and related theory, see the issue of *Brain and Cognition*, 262 (2), 1994.

3   The logical problem of the part and the whole is very ancient in both Eastern and Western civilizations. The reference book for the history of logic is still Kneale and Kneale (1962). It is interesting to know that the Polish logician Lesniewski built a formal system to deal with the "logic of parts". He called it "mereology" (from the greek *meros* = part). Perhaps someday we would need the neurological analog of mereology to give solid foundations to compensatory analysis. It is time to remember the importance given to the equilibrium and disequilibrium between parts and wholes in the early epistemological theory of Piaget (1918), Vidal (1994). It is also worthwhile remembering that Warren McCulloch (1965) the first neuroscientist to give a formal account of neural nets was perfectly aware of the problem of parts and wholes.

4   First schooling

1   I have recently proposed a fractal model of saccadic eye movements and a measure of the "temperature of sight," the "hotter" the visual exploration the higher the proportion of larger saccades (Battro, 1998, Mandelbrot, 1957, 1977). I would expect a "lower" temperature of sight as a consequence of Nico's hemianopia (a higher proportion of smaller – correcting – saccades). See also Rayner (1992).

6   The double brain

1   I thank my friend Marvin Minsky for his willingness to share his valuable views on the half-brained person. His cognitive theory is in Minsky (1987).

2   The study was carried out with 786 subjects on the tactile version of the Piagetian tasks and was performed in Brazil in several universities with the help of my collaborators: M. Bergamin, D. Cavicchia, S. Marchezi, A. Monteiro, I. Nogueira, M. Paiva, and O. Rembowski. I had the wonderful opportunity to discuss our results at one of the last seminars conducted by Jean Piaget at the Centre d'Episté-mologie Génétique in Geneva.

3   It is interesting to note that the Nobel prize in Medicine was awarded to two neuropsychologists, the Portuguese Egaz Monis who studied the leucotomized frontal lobe and the American Roger W. Sperry, who studied the split brain produced by callosotomy. In both cases neurosurgery altered the brain symmetry. The scientific literature on the topic is so enormous that here I shall only list some relevant books. For an evolutionary point of view see Benson and Zaidel 1985 and Corballis 1991.

   The works of Michel S. Gazzaniga alone suggest a whole program of research that started with the split brain studies: Gazzaniga (1970, 1978, 1985, 1997). The same can be said from the remarkable lateralization studies of the Harvard scientists Norman Geschwind and Alberto M. Galaburda (1987). For recent work see Davidson and Hugdahl (1995), Dimond and Blizard 1997), Iaccino (1993), Ivry and Robertson (1997).

7   Brain, education, and development

1   Piaget himself never studied the nervous system per se, but he recognized the impact of the neurosciences on the field of psychology in his book *Biologie et connaissance* (Piaget, 1967). Piaget was a biologist in the classical sense of a "naturaliste", he spent all his life working with two biological models, molluscs, *limneae*, and the small plants called *sedum*. Both were central to his research on the process of adaptation and evolution. In that book he dedicated one chapter to the nervous

system, emphasizing the correspondence between the neural networks of McCulloch-Pitts (1943) and the calculus of propositional logic in formal adolescent thinking. In the same vein I studied the isomorphisms between a McCulloch-Pitts neural model of the myotatic reflex and Piaget's INRC group in formal operations (Battro, 1977). The 1996 international conference in Geneva to celebrate the centenary of Piaget's birth was titled *The Growing Mind,* its logo was a brain and several of the more relevant papers were related to the neurosciences.

References

Adelson, P. D., Hovda, D. A., Villablanca, J. R. and Tatsukawa, K. (1995). Development of a crossed corticotectal pathway following cerebral hemispherectomy in cats: A quantitative study of the projecting neurons. *Brain Res. Dev.*, 86 (1–2), 81–93.

M. A. Arbib (ed.) (1995). *The handbook of brain theory and neuronal networks.* Cambridge, MA: MIT Press.

Austin, G., Hayward, W. and Rouhe, S. (1972). A note on the problem of conscious man and cerebral disconnection by hemispherectomy. In L. Smith (ed.) *Cerebral disconnection.* Springfield, Ill: C. Thomas Inc.

Bach y Rita, P. (1980). Brain plasticity as a basis for recovery of function in humans. *Neuropsychologia*, 28(6), 547–54.

Balasubramanian, V. (1997). Unilateral amygdalactomy and hemispherectomy. *Child's nervous system*, 13(3), 1211.

Basser, L. S. (1962). Hemiplegia of early onset and the faculty of speech with special reference to the effects of hemispherectomy. *Brain, 85*, 427–60.

Bates, E., Thai, D., Janowski, J. J. (1992). Early language development and its neural correlates. In J. J. Segalowitz and I. Rapin (eds.) *Handbook of neuropsychology*, 7. New York: Elsevier, pp. 69–110.

Battro, A. M. (1966). *Piaget dictionary of terms.* Oxford: Pergamon Press.

Battro, A. M. (1976). Morphogenèse des limnées, adaptation vitale et théorie des catastrophes. *Bulletin de Psychologie,* 30, 141–9.

Battro, A. M. (1976). Réflexions sur une psychologie écologique expérimentale. In G. Oléron (ed.) *Psychologie expérimentale et comparée: Hommage à Paul Fraisse.* Paris: Presses Universitaires de France.

Battro, A. M. (1977). Estructura de un circuito lógico elemental. Un modelo lógico de los reflejos miotáticos. *Estudos Cognitivos* (Univ. Est. S. Paulo, Araraquara), 1, 45–74.

Battro, A. M. (1981). Hemispheric lateralization in the development of spatial and logical reasoning in left and right-handed children. *Archives de Psychologie,* 49, 83–90.

Battro, A. M. and Ellis, P. J. (1989). *La imagen de la ciudad en los niños* (Unpublished Manuscript, Department of Urban Studies and Planning, MIT).

Battro, A. M. (1986). *Computación y aprendizaje especial: Aplicaciones del lenguaje Logo en el tratamiento de niños discapacitados.* Buenos Aires: El Ateneo.

Battro, A. M. and Denham, P. J. (1989). *Discomunicaciones: Computación y niños sordos.* Fundación Navarro Viola: Buenos Aires, El Ateneo. Trans. (1994). *Discomunicazioni: Tecnologia informatica ed educazione dei disabili uditivi.* Padova: Piccin.

Battro, A. M. (1991). Logo, talents et handicaps. In J. L. Gurtner and J. Retschitzki (eds.) *Logo et apprentissages.* Neuchâtel: Delachaux et Niestlé.

Battro, A. M. (1994). Intellectual Prostheses. Theory and Practice. *Pontificia Academia Scientiarum.* Plenary Session, October 25–29: The Vatican.

Battro, A. M.(1996). Le cerveau opératoire: Neurocognitive paths in psychological development. *The Growing Mind.* Symposium: Are Piaget's cognition models still valid? University of Geneva.

Battro, A. M. and Denham, P. J. (1997). *La educación digital.* Buenos Aires, Emecé. Trans. (1997). *Digital education:* www.byd.com.ar.

Battro, A. M. (1997). Half a brain is enough: A case study in neuroeducation. *7th International Conference On Thinking,* Singapore (June 1–6).

Battro, A. M. (1998). La temperatura de la mirada. In M. Guirao (ed.) *Procesos sensoriales y cognitivos: Artículos presentados en adhesión al 25 aniversario del Laboratorio de Investigaciones Sensoriales, Conicet.* Buenos Aires: Dunken.

Beardsworth, E. D. and Adams, C. B. T. (1988). Modified hemispherectomy for epilepsy: Early results in 10 cases. *British Journal of Neurosurgery,* 2, 73–84.

Benecke, R., Meyer, B. U. and Freund, H. J. (1991). Reorganization of descending motor pathways in patients after hemispherectomy and severe hemispheric lesions demonstrated by magnetic brain simulation. *Experimental Brain Research,* 83(2), 419–26.

Benson, F. D. and Zaidel, E. (1985). *The dual brain. Hemispheric specialization in humans.* New York: Guilford Press.

Bigler, E. D. (ed.) (1996). *Neuroimaging.* New York: Plenum.

Bickle, J. (1998). *Psychoneural reduction: The new wave.* Cambridge, MA: MIT Press.

Bisese, H. and Wang, A. (1994). *Pediatric cranial MRI: An atlas of neuronal development.* New York: Springer.

Bishop, D. V. M. (1983). Linguistic impairment after left hemidecortication for infantile hemiplegia. A reappraisal. *Quarterly Journal of Experimental Psychology, 35* A, 199–207.

Blinkov, S. M. and Glezer, I. I. (1968). The human brain in figures and tables. In M. A. Barzier and H. Petsche (eds.) *Architectonics of the cerebral cortex.* New York: Academic Press, pp. 443–65.

Borden, P. A., Fatherly, S., Ford, K. and Vanderheiden, G.C. (eds.) (1993–94). *Trace Resourcebook. Assistive Technologies for Communication, Control and Computer Access* (Waisman Center, University of Wisconsin-Madison. Madison), also: http://trace.wisc.edu/publications/1.html

Borod, J. C. (1992). Interhemispheric and intrahemispheric control of emotion: A focus on unilateral brain damage. *Journal of Consulting and Clinical Psychology, 60,* 339–48.

Burklund, C. W. and Smith, A. (1977). Language and the cerebral hemispheres: Observations of verbal and nonverbal responses during 18 months following left hemispherectomy. *Neurology, 27,* pp. 627, 633.

Byrne, J. and Gates, R. D. (1987). Single-case study of left cerebral hemispherectomy: Development in the first five years of life. *Journal of Clinical and Experimental Neuropsychology, 9*(4), 423–34.

Cardinali, D. P., Brusco, L. I., Selgasb, L. and Esquifino, A. I. (1997). Melatonin: A synchronizing signal for the immune system. *Neuroendocrinology Letters, 18,* 73–84.

Carmon, A. and Bechtold, H. P. (1973). Dominance of the right cerebral hemisphere for stereopsis. *Acta Psychologica, 37,* 351–7.

Chall, J. S. & Mirsky, A. F. (eds.) (1978). *Education and the brain,* Chicago University Press.

Changeux, J. P. (1981).*L'homme neuronal.* Paris: Gallimard. Trans. (1997). *Neuronal man. The biology of mind,* Princeton University Press.

Changeux, J. P. and Connes, A. (1992). *Matière à pensée.* Paris: Odile Jacob.

Changeux, J. P. and Ricoeur, P. (1998).*Ce qui nous fait penser: La Nature et la règle.* Paris: Odile Jacob.

Churchland, P. S. (1986). *Neurophilosophy: Toward a unified science of the mind-brain.* Cambridge, MA: MIT Press.

Churchland, P. M. (1996). *The engine of reason, the seat of the soul: A philosophical journey into the brain.* Cambridge, MA: MIT Press.

Claudel, P. (1957). *Oeuvres poétiques.* Paris: Gallimard.

Clark, A. (1996). *Being there: Putting brain, body, and world together again.* Cambridge, MA: MIT Press.

Corballis, M. C. (1983). *Human laterality.* New York: Academic Press.

Corballis, M. C. (1991). *The lopsided ape: Evolution of the generative mind.* New York: Oxford University Press.

Crick, F. (1994). *The astonishing hypothesis: The scientific search for the soul.* New York: Charles Scribner's Sons.

Damasio, A. R., Lima, A. and Damasio, H. (1975). Nervous function after right hemispherectomy. *Neurology, 25,* 89–93.

Damasio, A. and Damasio, H. (1989). *Lesion analysis in neuropsychology.* New York: Oxford University Press.

Damasio, A. R. (1994). *Descartes' error: Emotion, reason and the human brain.* New York: Avon.

Damasio, H. (1995). *Human brain anatomy in computerized images.* New York: Oxford University Press.

Dandy, W. E. (1928). Removal of right cerebral hemisphere for certain tumors with hemiplegia. *Journal of the American Medical Association, 90,* 823.

Davies, K. G, Maxwell, R. E. and French, L. A. (1993). Hemispherectomy for intractable seizures: long-term results in 17 patients followed for up to 38 years. *Journal of Neurosurgery, 78*(5), 733–40.

Davidson, R. J. and Hugdahl, K. (eds.) (1995). *Brain asymmetry.* Cambridge, MA: MIT Press.

Day, P. S. and Ulatowska, H. K. (1979). Perceptual, cognitive and linguistic development after early hemispherectomy: two case studies. *Brain and Language, 7,* 17–33.

Dehaene, S. (1997). *The number sense.* Oxford University Press.

Dehaene, S., Dupoux, E., Mehler, J., Cohen, L., Paulesu, E., Perani, D., Van de Moortele, P. F., Lehéricy, S. and Le Bihan, D. (1997). Anatomical variability in the cortical representation of first and second languages. *Neuroreport, 17,* 3775–8.

Dennis, M. and Kohn, B. (1975). Comprehension of syntax in infantile hemiplegics after cerebral hemidecortication. *Brain and Language, 10,* 287–317.

Dennis, M. and Whitaker, H. A. (1976). Language acquisition following hemidecortication. Linguistic superiority of the left over the right hemisphere. *Brain and Language, 3,* 404–33.

Dennis, M. and Whitaker, H. A. (1977). Hemispheric equipotentiality and language acquisition. In J. Segalowitz and F. Gruber (eds.) *Language development and neurological theory*. New York: Academic Press.

Dennis, M. (1980). Capacity and strategy for syntactic comprehension after left or right hemidecortication. *Brain and Langage*, 10, 287–317.

Dennis, M., Lovett, M. and Wiegel-Crump, C.A. (1981). Written language acquisition after left or right decortication in infancy. *Brain and Language*, 12, 54–91.

Dennet, D. C. (1991). *Consciousness explained*. Boston: Little Brown.

Deonna, T. (1998). Developmental consequences of epilepsies in infancy. In A. Nenling, J. Motte, S. L. Moshe and P. Plovin. *Childhood epilepsies and brain development*. London: John Libbey Publishers.

Dickinson, E. (1978). *Complete poems*. T. H. Johnson (ed.) Boston: Little Brown.

Dimond, S. J. and Blizard, D. A. (eds.) (1997). *Evolution and lateralization of the brain*. New York Academy of Sciences, vol. 299.

Donaldson, H. H. (1896). *The growth of the brain: A study of the nervous system in relation to education*. London: Scribner's & Sons.

Edelman, C. M. and Mountcastle, V. B. (1978). *The mindful brain*. Cambridge, MA: MIT Press.

Edelman, G. M. (1992). *Bright air, brillant fire*. New York: Basic Books.

Epstein, H. T. (1974). Phrenoblysis: Special brain and mind growth periods. *Developmental Psychobiology*, 7, 207–16, 217–24.

Epstein, H. T. (1979). Correlated brain and intelligence development in humans. In M. H. Hahn, C. Jensen and B. C. Dudek (eds.) *Development and evolution of brain size: Behavioral implications*. New York: Academic Press.

Epstein, H. T. (1978). Growth spurts during brain development: Implications for educational policy and practice. In J. S. Chall and A. F. Mirsky (eds.) (1978).

Evrad, O. and Minkowski, A. (1989). *Developmental neurobiology*. New York: Raven Press.

Fischer, K. W. and Rose, S. P. (1994). Dynamic development of coordination of components in brain and behavior: A framework for theory and research. In G. Dawson and K. W. Fischer (eds.) *Human behavior and the developing brain*. New York: Guilford, pp. 3–66.

Fischer, K. W. and Rose, S. P. (1996). Dynamic growth cycles of brain and cognitive development. In R. Thatcher, G. R. Lyon, J. Rumsey and N. Krasnegor (eds.) *Developmental neuroimaging. Mapping the development of brain and behavior*. New York: Academic Press.

Fischer, K. W. and Bidell, T. R. (1998). Dynamic development of psychological structures in action and thought.

A. Damon and R. M. Lerner (eds.) *Handbook of child psychology*, vol. 1. New
York: Wiley.

Franco, L. and Sperry, R. W. (1977). Hemispheric specialization for cognitive processing of geometry. *Neuropsychologia*, 15, 107–14.

Frégnac, Y. (1998). Hebbian synaptic plasticity: Comparative and developmental
aspects. In M. A. Arbib, P. Erdi, and J. Szentágothai (eds.) *Neural organization*,
Cambridge, MA: MIT Press.

Gainotti, G. (1972). Emotional behavior and hemispheric side of the lesion. *Cortex*,
8, 41–55.

Gardner, W. J. (1933). Removal of the right cerebral hemisphere for infiltrating
glioma. *Journal of the American Medical Association*, 101, 823–6.

Gardner, H. (1982). *Art, mind and brain: A cognitive approach to creativity*. New
York: Basic Books.

Gardner, H., Brownell, H. H., Wapner, W. and Michelow, D. (1983). Missing the
point: The role of the right hemisphere in the processing of complex linguistic
materials. In E. Pericman (ed.) *Cognitive processes and the right hemisphere*.
New York: Academic Press.

Gardner, H. (1985). *Frames of mind: the theory of multiple intelligences*. New York:
Basic Books.

Gardner, H. (1991). *The unschooled mind: How children think and how schools
should teach*. New York: Basic Books.

Gardner, H. (1993). *Multiple intelligences: The theory in practice*. New York: Basic
Books.

Gardner, H. (1999). *Intelligence reframed: Multiples intelligences for the 21st
century*. New York: Basic Books.

Gazzaniga, M. S. (1970). *The bisected brain*. New York: Appleton.

Gazzaniga, M. (1978). *The integrated mind*. New York: Plenum.

Gazzaniga, M. S. (1985). *The social brain: Discovering the networks of the mind*.
New York: Basic Books.

Gazzaniga, M. S. (1985). *Mind matters. How mind and brain interact to create our
conscious life*. Boston: Houghton Mifflin.

Gazzaniga, M. S. (ed.) (1995). *The cognitive neurosciences*. Cambridge, MA: MIT
Press.

Gazzaniga, M. S. (ed.) (1997). *Conversations in the cognitive neurosciences*. Cambridge, MA: MIT Press.

Geshwind, N. and Galaburda, A. (1987). *Cerebral lateralization*. Cambridge, MA: Harvard University Press.

Gibson, E. and Levin, H. (1985). *The psychology of reading*. Cambridge, MA: MIT Press.

Gilles, F. H., Levinton, A. and Dooling, E. C. (1983). *The developing human brain: Growth and epidemiologic neuropathology*. Boston: John Wright.

Goldman-Rakic, P. and Rakic, P. (1984). Experimental modification of gyral patterns. In N. Geschwind and A. M. Galaburda (eds.) *Cerebral dominance: The biological foundations*. Cambridge, MA: Harvard University Press.

Goldman-Rakic, P. (1987). Development of cortical circuitry and cognitive function. *Child Development*, 58, 601–22.

Goldstein, K. (1940). *Human nature in the light of psychopathology*. Cambridge, MA: Harvard University Press.

Goldstein, K. (1934). *Der Aufbau des Organismus*. Haag: Nijhoff, Trans. (1995) *The organism*. New York: Zone Books.

Gould, S. J. (1981). *The mismeasure of man*. New York: Norton.

Gott, P. S. (1973). Cognitive abilities following right and left hemispherectomy. *Cortex*, 9, 266–74.

Gott, P. S. (1973). Language after dominant hemispherectomy. *Journal of Neurology, Neurosurgery and Psychiatry*, 36, 1082–8.

Graham, G. and Lynn Stephens, G. (eds.) (1997). *Philosophical psychopathology*. Cambridge, MA: MIT Press.

Gray, D. B. and Kavanagh, F. (eds.) (1985). *Biobehavioral measures of dyslexia*. New York: York Press.

Green, R. C., Adler, J. R. and Erba, G. (1988) Epilepsy surgery in children. *Journal of Child Neurology*, 3(3), 155–66.

Greenough, W. T. (1986). What's special about development? Thoughts on the bases of experience-sensitive synaptic plasticity. In W. T. Greenough and J. M. Juraska (eds.) *Developmental neuropsychology*. New York: Academic Press, pp. 387–407.

Haier, R. J, Siegel, B. V., MacLachlan, A., Soderling, E., Lottenberg, S. and Buchsbaum, M. S. (1992). Regional cerebral glucose metabolic changes after learning a complex visuospatial/motor task: A positron emission tomographic study. *Brain Research*, 570, 134–43.

Hanlon, R. E. (1991). *Cognitive microgenesis: A neuropsychological perspective*. New York: Springer Verlag.

Harris, L. J. (1988). Right-brain training: Some reflections on the application of research on cerebral hemispheric specialization to education. In L. F. Molfese and

S. J. Segalowitz (eds.) *Brain lateralization in children*. New York: The Guilford Press, pp. 207–35.

Hatwell, Y., Stephens, B. and Verder, P. (1985). *Piaget reasoning and the blind*. American Foundation for the Blind.

Heilman, K., Watson, R. T., and Bowers, D. (1983). Affective disorders associated with hemispheric disease. In K. Heilman and P. Satz (eds.) *Neuropsychology of human emotion*. New York: The Guilford Press.

Homer. *The Odyssey*. R. Fagles (Trans.). (1997). New York: Penguin Books.

Hudspeth, W. J. and Pribram, K. H. (1990). Stages of brain and cognitive maturation. *Journal of Educational Psychology*, 82, 881–4.

Hudspeth, W. J. and Pribram, K. H. (1991). Physiological indices of cerebral maturation. *International Journal of Psychophysiology*, 12, 19–29.

Huttenlocher, P. R. (1984). Synapse elimination and plasticity in developing human cerebral cortex. *American Journal of Mental Deficiency*, 88, 488–95.

Huttenlocher, P. R. (1990). Morphometric study of human cerebral cortex development. *Neuropsychologia*, 28, 517–27.

Iaccino, J. F. (1993). *Left brain – Right brain differences*. New Jersey: Erlbaum.

Ivry, R. B. and Robertson, L. C., (1997). *The two sides of perception*. Cambridge, MA: MIT Press.

Jerison, H. J. (1979). The evolution and diversity in brain size. In M. E. Hahn, C. Jensen and B. C. Dudek (eds.) *Development and evolution of brain size: Behavioral implications*. New York: Academic Press.

Jerison, H. J. (1997). The theory of encephalization. In D. A. Blizard (ed.) *Evolution and lateralization of the brain*. New York Academy of Sciences, pp. 146–58.

Julesz, B. (1971). *Foundations of cyclopean perception*. University of Chicago Press.

King, S. M., Frey, S., Villemure, J. G., Ptito, A. and Azzopardi, P. (1996). Perception of motion-in-depth in patients with partial or complete cerebral hemispherectomy. *Behavioural Brain Research*. 76(1–2), 169–80.

Kipling, R. (1927). *Rudyard Kipling verse*. London: Hodder.

Kneale, W. and Kneale M. (1962). *The development of logic*. Oxford: Clarendon Press.

Koch, C. and Davis J. L. (eds.) (1994). *Large-scale neuronal theories of the brain*. Cambridge, MA: MIT Press.

Kohn, B. and Dennis, M. (1974). Selective impairments of visual-spatial abilities in infantile hemiplegics after right cerebral hemidecortication. *Neuropsychologia*, 12, 505–12.

Kohn, B. and Dennis, M. (1974). Patterns of hemispheric specialization after hemidecortication for intractable hemiplegics. In M. Kinsbourne and W. Lynne-Smith
(eds.) *Hemispheric disconnection and cerebral function.* Springfield: Thomas.

Kosslyn, S. M. and van Kleeck, M. (1990). Broken brains and normal minds: Why
Humpty-Dumpty needs a skeleton. In E. L. Schwartz (ed.) *Computational neuroscience.* Cambridge, MA: MIT Press.

Kosslyn, S. and Koenig, O. (1992). *Wet mind: The new cognitive neuroscience.* New
York: Free Press.

Krynauw, R. A. (1950). Infantile hemiplegia treated by removing one cerebral hemisphere. *Journal of Neurology, Neurosurgery and Psychology,* 13, 243–67.

Lampl, M. and Emde, R. M. (1983). Episodic growth in infancy. A preliminary
report on length, head circumference, and behavior. In K. W. Fisher (ed.) *Levels
and transitions in children's development: New directions for child development,*
21, 21–36. San Francisco: Jossey-Bass.

Lampl, M., Veldhuis, J. D. and Johnson, M. L. (1992). Saltation and stasis: A model
of human growth. *Science,* 258, 801–803.

Lebrun, Y., van Endert, C. and Szliwowski, H. (1988). Trilingual hyperlexia. In L. K.
Obler and D. Fein (eds.) *The exceptional brain: Neuropsychology of talent and
special abilities.* New York: The Guilford Press.

Lenneberg, F. H. (1967). *Developmental foundations of language.* New York: Wiley.

Lezak, M. D. (1995). *Neuropsychological assessment.* New York: Oxford University
Press.

L'Hermite, J. (1928). L'ablation complète de l'hemisphère droit dans le cas de
tumeur cérébrale localisée compliquée d'hémiplégie. La décérébration surthala-
mique unilatérale chez l'homme. *L'Encéphale,* 23, 314–23.

Lindsay, J., Ounsted, C. and Richards, P. (1987). Hemispherectomy for childhood
epilepsy: A 36 year study. *Developmental Medicine and Child Neurology,* 29,
592–600.

Lister, R. (1995). Fractal strategies for neural networking scaling. In M. A. Arbib
(ed.) *The handbook of brain theory and neuronal networks.* Cambridge, MA:
MIT Press.

Luria, A. R. (1972). *The man with a shattered world: The history of a brain wound*
(with a foreword by O. Sacks). Cambridge, MA: Harvard University Press.

Luria, A. R. (1986). *The making of mind. A personal account of soviet psychology.*
Cambridge, MA: Harvard University Press.

Luria, A. R. (1988). *The mind of a mnemonist: A little book about a vast memory*
(with a foreword by Jerome Bruner),Cambridge, MA: Harvard University Press.

Lynch, K. (1960). *The image of the city*. Cambridge, MA: MIT Press.

Lynch, K. (ed.) (1979). *Growing up in cities*. Cambridge, MA: MIT Press.

Mandelbrot, B. B. (1957). Linguistique statistique macroscopique. In J. Piaget, L. Apostel, B. B. Mandelbrot and A. Morf (eds.) *Etudes d' épistémologie génétique: Logique, langage et théorie de l'information*. Paris: Presses Universitaires de France.

Mandelbrot, B. B. (1977). *Fractals, form, chance and dimension*. San Francisco: Freeman.

Merleau-Ponty, M. (1942). *La structure du comportement*. Paris: Presses Universitaires de France. Trans. (1963). *The structure of behavior*. Boston: Beacon Press.

Merleau-Ponty, M. (1944). *La phénoménologie de la perception*. Paris: Gallimard. Trans. (1976). *Phenomenology of perception*. London: Routledge & Kegan Paul.

McCulloch, W. S. and Pitts, W. S. (1943). A logical calculus of the ideas immanent in nervous activity. *Bull. Math. Biophysics*, 5, 115–13.

McCulloch, W. S. (1965). *Embodiments of mind*. Cambridge, MA: MIT Press.

McKenzie, K. G. (1938). The present status of a patient who has a right hemisphere removed. *Journal of the American Medical Association*. 111, 168.

McFie, J. (1961). The effects of hemispherectomy on intellectual functioning in cases of infantile hemiplegia. *Journal of Neurology, Neurosurgery and Psychiatry*, 24, 240–9.

Minsky, M. (1987). *The society of mind*. New York: Simon & Schuster.

Minsky, M. and Harrison, H. (1993). *The Turing option*. New York: Wraner Books.

Morrison, P., Morrison P. and the Office of Charles and Ray Eames (1994). *Powers of ten: About the relative size of things in the universe*. San Franciso, CA: Freeman.

Müller, F., Kunesh, E., Bikofski, F. and Freund, H. J. (1991). Residual sensorimotor functions in a patient after right-sided hemispherectomy. *Neuropsychologia*, 29(2), 125–45.

Nowinski, W. L., Fang, A., Nguyen, B. T., Raphel, J. K., Jagannathan, L., Raghavan, R., Bryn, R. N. and Miller, G. A. (1997). Multiple brain atlas database and atlas-based neuroimaging system. *Computer Aided Surgery*, 2, 42–66.

Obrador, S. (1964). Nervous integration after hemispherectomy in man. In G. Shaltenbrand and C. N. Woosley (eds.) *Cerebral localization and organization*. Madison: University of Wisconsin Press, pp. 133–54.

Odgen, J. A. (1988). Language and memory functions after long recovery periods in left-hemispherectomized subjects. *Neuropsychologia*, 26(5), 645–59.

Papert, S. (1961). Centrally produced geometrical illusion. *Nature*, 191, 733.

Papert, S. and Weir, S. (1978). Information prosthetics for the handicapped, *Artificial Intelligence Memo 496*. Cambridge, MA: MIT Press.

Papert, S. (1980). *Mindstorms. Children, computers and powerful ideas*. Cambridge, MA: MIT Press.

Papert, S. (1997). *The connected family*. New York: Basic Books.

Patterson, K., Vargha-Khadem, F. and Polkey, C. E. (1989). Reading with one hemisphere. *Brain*, 112, 39–63.

Pawlick, G., Holthoff, V. A., Kessler, J., Rudolf, J., Hebold, I. R., Lottgen, J. and Heiss, W. D. (1990). Positron emission tomography findings relevant to neurosurgery for epilepsy. *Acta Neurochir. Suppl. Wien*, 50, 84–7.

Peacock, W. J., Wehby-Grant, M. C., Shields, W. D., Shewmon, D. A., Chugani, H. T. and Sankar, B. (1996). Hemispherectomy for intractable seizures in children: a report of 58 cases. *Child's Nervous System*, 12(7), 376–84.

Piaget, J. (1918). *Recherche*. Lausanne: La Concorde.

Piaget, J. (1936). *La naissance de l'intelligence chez l enfant*. Neuchâtel: Delachaux et Niestlé. Trans. (1952). *The origins of intelligence in children*. New York: International University Press.

Piaget, J. (1937). *La construction du réel chez l'enfant*. Neuchâtel: Delachaux et Niestlé. Trans. (1954). *The construction of reality in the child*, New York: Basic Books.

Piaget, J. and Inhelder, B. (1941). *Le développement des quantités chez l'enfant*. Neuchâtel: Delachaux et Niestlé. Trans. (1974) *The child's construction of quantities. Conservation and atomism*. London: Routledge and Kegan Paul.

Piaget, J. and Szeminska, A. (1941). *La genèse du nombre chez l'enfant*. Paris: Presses Universitaires de France. Trans. (1965). *The child's conception of number*. London: Routledge & Kegan Paul.

Piaget, J. (1945). *La formation du symbole chez l' enfant*. Neuchâtel: Delachaux et Niestlé. Trans. (1962). *Play, dreams and imitation in childhood*. New York: Norton.

Piaget, J. and Inhelder, B. (1947). *La représentation de l'espace chez l'enfant*. Paris: Presses Universitaires de France. Trans. (1967). *The child's conception of space*. New York: W. W. Norton.

Piaget, J., Inhelder, B. and Szeminska, A. (1948). *La géométrie spontanée de l'enfant*. Paris: Presses Universitaires de France. Trans. (1981). *The child's concept of geometry*. New York: Norton.

Piaget, J. (1950). *Introduction à l'épistémologie génétique. vol. I. La pensée mathématique*. Paris: Presses Universitaires de France.

Piaget, J. and Inhelder, B. (1956). *La genèse de l'idée de hasard chez l'enfant*. Paris:

Presses Universitaires de France. Trans. (1975). *The origin of the idea of chance in children.* London: Routledge & Kegan Paul.

Piaget, J. (1957). L'actualité de Jean Amos Comenius. In *Jean Amos Comenius, 1592–1670. Pages choisies.* pp. 11–33, Paris: Unesco. Trans. (1967). *John Amos Comenius on education.* New York: Teachers College.

Piaget, J. (1961). *Les mécanismes perceptifs: Modèles probabilistes, analyse génétique, relations avec l'intelligence.* Paris: Presses Universitaires de France. Trans. (1969). *The mechanisms of perception.* London: Routledge & Kegan Paul, New York: Basic Books.

Piaget, J. and Inhelder, B. (1963). Les opérations intellectuelles et leur développement. In P. Fraisse and J. Piaget (eds.) *Traité de Psychologie Expérimentale.* Paris: Presses Universitaires de France. Trans. (1969). *Experimental psychology: Its scope and method. Intelligence.* vol. 7. London: Routledge & Kegan Paul.

Piaget, J. and Inhelder, B. (1966). *L'image mentale chez l'enfant.* Paris: Presses Universitaires de France.

Piaget, J. (1967). *Biologie et connaissance. Essai sur les relations entre les régulations organiques et les processus cognitifs.* Paris: Gallimard. Trans. (1971). *Biology and knowledge: An essay on the relations between organic regulations and cognitive processes.* University of Chicago Press.

Piaget, J. (1975). *L'équilibration des structures cognitives: Problème central du développement.* Paris: Presses Universitaires de France. Trans. (1985). *Equilibration of cognitive structures.* University of Chicago Press.

Piatelli-Palmarini, M. (1993). *L'illusioni di sapere.* Milano: Mondadori.

Piatelli-Palmarini, M. (ed.) (1979). *Théories du langage, théories de l'apprentissage: Le débat entre Jean Piaget et Noam Chomsky.* Paris: Seuil. Trans. (1980). *Language and learning: The debate between Jean Piaget and Noam Chomsky.* Cambridge, MA: Harvard University Press.

Piatelli-Palmarini, M. (1994). Ever since language and learning: Afterthoughts on the Piaget-Chomsky debate. *Cognition,* 50, 315–46.

Plaut, D. (1995). Lesioned attractor networks as models of neuropsychological deficits. In M. A. Arbib (ed.) *The handbook of brain theory and neural networks.* Cambridge, MA: MIT Press.

Poirier, P., Lassonde, M., Villemure, J. G., Geoffroy, G. and Lepore, F. (1994). Sound localization in hemispherectomized patients. *Neuropsychologia,* 32(5), 541–53.

Popper, K. (1965). *The logic of scientific discovery.* New York: Harper (2 ed).

Popper, K. R. and Eccles, J. (1977). *The self and its brain: An argument for interac-*

tionism. New York: Springer.

Posner, M. I. and Raichle, M. E. (1994). *Images of mind*, New York: Scientific American.

Rabinowicz, T. (1979). The differentiate maturation of the human cerebral cortex. In F. Falkner and J. Tanner (eds.) *Human growth. Neurobiology and nutrition*, New York: Plenum Press, pp. 97–123.

Rasmussen, T. (1983). Hemispherectomy for seizures revisited. *Canadian Journal of Neurol. Science*, 10, 71–8.

Rasmussen, T. and Villemure, J. G. (1989). Cerebral hemispherectomy for seizures with hemiplegia. *Cleveland Clinical Journal of Medicine*, 56, 562–8.

Rayner, K. (ed.) (1992). *Eye movements and visual cognition*. New York: Springer Verlag.

Reggini, H. C. (1985). *Ideas y formas: Explorando el espacio con Logo*. Buenos Aires: Ediciones Galápago.

Renouz, G. (1988). The cortex relates the immune system and the activities of the T-cell specific immune potentiator. *International Journal of Neuroscience*, 39, 177–87.

Rosenzweig, M. (1979). Responsiveness of brain size to individual experience, behavioral and evolutionary implications. In M. E. Hahn, C. Jensen and B. C. Dudek (eds.) *Development and evolution of brain size: Behavioral implications*. New York Academy of Sciences.

Rozestraten, R. A., Battro, A. M. and Santos Andrade, A. (1976). A visual catastrophe: The reversal of the Oppel Kundt illusion in the open field. *Actes du XXI Congrès de Psychologie*, Paris.

Saban, R. (1995). Image of the human fossil brain: Endocranial cast and meningeal vessels in young and adult subjects. In J. P. Changeux and J. Chavaillon (eds.) *Origins of the human brain*. Oxford: Clarendon Press.

Sacks, O. (1987). *The man who mistook his wife for a hat, and other clinical tales*. New York: Harper & Row.

Sacks, O. (1995). *An anthropologist on Mars: Seven paradoxical tales*. New York: Knopf.

Sacks, O. (1997). *The island of the color blind and Cycad Island*. New York: Knopf.

Salamon, G., Raynaud, C., Regis, J. and Rumeau, C. (1990). *Magnetic resonance imaging of the pediatric brain*. New York: Raven Press.

Satz, P. A. (1979). Test of some models of hemispheric speech organization in left and right-handed. *Science*, 203, 1131–3.

Schacter, S. C. and Devinsky, O. (eds.) (1997). *Behavioral neurology and the legacy of*

Norman Geschwind. New York: Lippincot-Raven.

Schütz, A. (1995). Neuroanatomy in a computational perspective. In M. A. Arbib (ed.) *The handbook of brain theory and neuronal networks*. Cambridge, MA: MIT Press.

Sergent, J. and Villemure, J. G. (1989). Prosopagnosia in a right hemispherectomized patient. *Brain*, 112, 975–95.

Silbersweig, D. A., Stern, E., Frith, C., Cahill, C., Holmes, A., Groontoonk, S., Seaward, J., McKenna, P., Chua, S. E., Schnorr, l., Jones, T. and Frackowiack, R. S. J. (1995). A functional neuroanatomy of hallucinations in schizophrenia. *Nature*, 378, 176–9.

Simon, H. A. (1981). *The sciences of the artificial*. Cambridge, MA: MIT Press (2 ed).

Smith, A. (1974) Dominant and nondominant hemispherectomy. In M. Kinsbourne and W. L. Smith (eds.) *Hemispheric disconnection and cerebral function*. Springfield. Ill.: Thomas, pp. 5–33.

Smith, A. and Sugar, O. (1975). Development of above-normal language and intelligence twenty one years after left hemispherectomy. *Neurology*, 25, 813–18.

Smith, S. J., Anderman, F., Villemure, J. G., Rasmussen, T. B. and Quesney, L. F. (1991). Functional hemispherectomy: EEG findings, spiking from isolated brain postoperatively and prediction of outcome. *Neurology*, 41(11), 1790–4.

Stark, R. E., Blesjle, K. M., Brandt, J., Vining, E. P. G. and Freeman, J. (1995). Speech-language outcomes of hemispherectomy in children and young adults. *Brain and Language*, 51, 406–21.

Stark, R. E. and McGregor, K. K. (1997). Follow-up study of a right and a left-hemispherectomized child. Implications for localization and impairment of language in children. *Brain and Language*, 66, 222–43.

Stein, P. S. G., Selverston, A. I. and Stuart, D. G. (eds.) (1998). *Neurons, networks, and motor behavior*. Cambridge, MA: MIT Press.

Swerdlow, J. L. (1995). Quiet miracles of the brain. *National Geographic Magazine*, June, pp. 5–41.

Solso, R. L. (ed.) (1997). *Mind and brain sciences in the 21st century*. Cambridge, MA: MIT Press.

Terman, L. M. and Oden, M. H. (1959). *Genetic studies of genius, vol . 5. The gifted group at mid-life: Thirty-five years' follow-up of the superior child*. Stanford, CA: Stanford University Press.

Thatcher, R. W. (1994). Cyclic cortical reorganization. Origins of human cognitive development. In G. Dawson and K. W. Fischer (eds.) *Human behavior and the developing brain*. New York: The Guilford Press.

Tinuper, F., Andermann, F., Villemure, J. G., Rasmussen, T. B. and Quesney, L. F.

(1988). Functional hemispherectomy for treatment of epilepsy associated with hemiplegia: rationale, indications, results, and comparisons with callosotomy. *Annals of Neurology*, 24 (1), 27–34.

Thom, R. (1972). *Stabilité structurale et morphogenèse*. Paris: Ediscience. Trans. (1989). *Structural stability and morphogenesis. Outline of a general theory of models*. New York: Addison Wesley.

Thompson, D. W. (1952). *On growth and form*. Cambridge University Press.

Tversky, A. and Kahneman, D. (1982). *Judgment under uncertainty: Heuristics and biases*. New York: Cambridge University Press.

Valente, J. (1983). Creating a computer-based learning environment for physically handicapped children. (Unpublished doctoral dissertation. Department of Mechanical Engineering: MIT).

Vargha-Khadem, F. and Polkey, C. E. (1992). A review of cognitive outcome after hemidecortication in humans. In F. D. Rose and D. A. Johnson (eds.) *Recovery from brain damage*. New York: Plenum.

Vargha-Khadem, F., Isaacs, E. B., Papaleloudi, H., Polkey, C. E. and Wilson, J. (1991). Development of language in six hemispherectomized patients. *Brain*, 114, 473–95.

Verity, C. M., Strauss, E. H., Moyes, P. B., Wada, J. A., Dunn, H. G. and La Pointe, J. S. (1982). Long-term follow up after cerebral hemispherectomy: neurophysiological, radiologic and psychological findings. *Neurology*, 32, 629–39.

Villemure, J. G. and Rasmussen, T. B. (1993). Functional hemispherectomy in children. *Neuropediatrics*, 24(1), 53–5.

Villemure, J. G. and Mascott, C. R. (1995). Peri-insular hemispherectomy: Surgical principles and anatomy. *Neurosurgery*, 37(5), 975–81.

Waddington, C. H. (1974). A catastrophe theory of evolution. *Ann. New York Academy of Sciences*, 231, 32–42.

Wang, X. and Blum, E. K. (1995). Dynamics and bifurcation of neural networks. In M. A. Arbib (ed.) *The handbook of brain theory and neuronal networks*. Cambridge, MA: MIT Press.

Webster's Ninth New Collegiate Dictionary. (1991). New York: Merrian Webster.

Wilson, P. J. E. (1970). Cerebral hemispherectomy for infantile hemiplegia: A report of 50 cases. *Brain*, 93, 147–80.

Whitaker, H. A. and Ojeman, G. (1977). Lateralization of higher cortical functions: A critique. In S. F. Diamond & D. A. Blizard (eds.) *Evolution and lateralization of the brain. Ann. New York Academy of Sciences*, 299, 459–73.

White, H. H. (1961). Cerebral hemispherectomy in the treatment of infantile hemiplegia: Review of the literature and report of two cases. *Confinia Neurologica*, Basel, 21, 1–50.

Winner, E. (1996). *Gifted children: Myths and realities*. New York: Basic Books.

Zaidel, E. (1973). Linguistic competence and related functions in the right cerebral hemisphere of man following commissurotomy and hemispherectomy. *California Institute of Technology, Thesis*. Pasadena, California.

Zaidel, E. (1980). The split and half-brain as models of congenital language disability. In C. L. Ludlow and M. E. Doran-Quine (eds.) *The neurological basis of language disorders in children: Methods and directions for research*. Bethesda: NIH.

Zaidel, E. (1981). Language in the right hemisphere. In D. F. Benson and E. Zaidel (eds.) *The dual brain: Hemispheric specialization in humans*. New York: The Guilford Press, pp. 205–31.

Index